the healing aromatherapy bath

Therapeutic Treatments
Using Meditation,
Visualization
& Essential Oils

Margó Valentine Lazzara

STOREY
BOOKS

The mission of Storey Communications is to serve our customers by publishing practical information that encourages personal independence in harmony with the environment.

Edited by Deborah Balmuth and Robin Catalano
Cover and text design by Betty Kodela
Cover photograph by Shahram Sanai/The Stock Market
Photos styled by Betty Kodela
Photographs by PhotoDisc, Inc., except floral photos by Giles Prett
Text production by Jennifer Jepson Smith
Indexed by Peggy Holloway, Holloway Indexing Services
Professional review by Donna Maria Coles

The information in this book is true and complete to the best of our knowledge. All recommendations are made without guarantee on the part of the author or Storey Books. The author and publisher disclaim any liability in connection with the use of this information. For additional information, please contact Storey Books, Schoolhouse Road, Pownal, Vermont 05261.

Storey books are available for special premium and promotional uses and for customized editions. For further information, please call Storey's Custom Publishing Department at 1-800-793-9396.

Printed in Canada by Transcontinental Printing
10 9 8 7 6 5 4 3 2 1

Library of Congress Cataloging-in-Publication Data

Lazzara, Margó Valentine, 1955-
    The healing aromatherapy bath : therapeutic treatments using meditation, visualization, and essential oils / Valentine Lazzara.
        p.   cm.
    Includes index.
    ISBN 1-58017-197-4 (pbk.)
    1. Aromatherapy.   2. Baths.   3. Stress management.   I. Title.
RM666.A68L396   1999
615'.321—dc21
                                                                99-29330
                                                                    CIP

Dedication

This book is a tribute to my mother, Marin, in Heaven,
who was responsible for instilling determination and
strong values in my upbringing.
She was a beautiful woman, full of wisdom, devotion, love,
tenderness, and strength all at the same time.
My mother taught me the magic splendor of flowers and prayer.
She helped me see the beauty in all things and in all people.
She is my constant source of spiritual inspiration.

~

And to my wonderful husband and soul mate, Sebastian,
who gives me encouragement and support in all my endeavors,
and showers me with a love that is filled with all the vibrant colors
of the rainbow.

Acknowledgments

Abundant thanks to Steven Rosenfeld, my agent and manager, who planted in my mind the seed of this book and made this dream come to fruition. He was instrumental in making it all happen.

Sincere gratitude to everyone at Storey Books, especially my editors, Deborah Balmuth and Robin Catalano. Special thanks to Robin Allen-Payne for typing and proofreading, and for being the best writer's assistant I ever could have wished for.

Loving thanks to my mother-in-law and father-in-law, Maria and Nino Lazzara, for their love and support with this project, for accepting me into their family, and for loving and spoiling me like their own daughter. Loving thanks also to my sister, Luz Maria Crespo, whose prayers and blessings have been inspirational.

Warm thanks to Jean Moné for being a friend, publicly acknowledging my potential on her radio and TV shows, and believing in my Aromatica aromatherapy products. And thank-you to Nancy Thomas, for mailing me every aromatherapy book she could find throughout the years.

Thanks to Gary DiToro, of Arden Studios, Inc., on Staten Island, New York for publicity photo shoots, to Dr. Stephen T. Mastrianni for his *JAMA* research, and to Reverend Charmaine Colon for her spiritual guidance and encouragement in completing this book.

Grateful thanks to Sylvana C. Lazzara, Lisa DeRosa, and my cousin Sonia Irizarry in Puerto Rico for their unlimited research contributions.

Thanks to Jeanne Jacobs for being a loving friend and inspiring artistic creativity. I also thank Danny, Dawn, and Tony Lazzara and Cara Perrotta in helping me get this project off the ground despite my lack of computer skills, and my cousins Jane Lodato and Helen Mastrianni for unlimited loving encouragement.

Thank you to Dr. John Ziegler of the Ziegler Institute in New York City for his mentoring and training in Gestalt therapy and referring patients to start my practice, and to my professors at New York University for discipline, encouragement, and wisdom.

Heartfelt thanks to Dr. Michael Ellner, President of H.E.A.L. (Health Education and AIDS Liaison) in New York City, who started me on the rewarding journey of providing healing circles for those with weakened immune systems. Thank you also to all the patients who allowed me to try new treatments with them.

And most of all, thanks to God for the unconditional love, strength, and happiness that he has given me throughout my life.

Contents

Preface

Welcome to the powerful world of scent! My name is Margó Valentine Lazzara. I am a certified clinical hypnotherapist and aromatherapist, and I have been using aromatherapy with hypnosis successfully for ten years. Allow me to give you a brief history on how all of this started.

As a child, I was strongly influenced by my mother's homeopathic use of poultices made of plants, vegetables, and oils found in our kitchen. Her recipes and secrets were passed down through the generations of our Puerto Rican Indian ancestors. Any scrapes, bruises, fevers, and tummy aches were effectively remedied in this manner. Even my bathwater was magically transformed with carnation petals, plants, floral waters, and oils.

Spiritual reflection and introspection were encouraged and guided during this time. It was a gift that my mother lovingly gave to me throughout her life. It encouraged strength, faith, inner peace, emotional and spiritual growth, and a certain curiosity about the spiritual mystery of flowers. I grew up feeling that each flower had its own "soul" and I soon found out that each does have its own unique properties.

My interest resurfaced when I started using essential oils to stimulate the olfactory pathways in the brain to elicit a variety of specific feelings, emotions, and moods in conjunction with my hypnosis sessions. The effects of essential oils can last for days, and because of the link with the emotional centers of the brain, a subtle scent can leave an impression for a lifetime.

For many years, the seeds of this book had germinated in the most fertile parts of my mind. The most lovely garden started to grow and blossom. I now share with you the abundance of its beauty for healing the body, the mind, and the soul. An open mind and heart plus the desire to enrich your life are all you need to bring to this book — then prepare yourself for some rather startling and truly wonderful results!

This is an instructional book on the use and creation of essential oil blends for getting in touch with your inner self, along with guided imagery, meditation, and visualization to stimulate and awaken the senses and to heal the body, mind, and spirit. Included are recipe blends that will transform your bathwater and create a healthy state of mind receptive to positive suggestions, guided imagery, and affirmations. All of them are uncomplicated, precise, and enjoyable even for the novice.

The exercises will help eliminate the daily stress caused by our fast-paced society. Negative stress comes from a variety of sources: work, family life, unexpected change, loss of job, financial problems, and sexual problems, to name just a few. The immune system is weakened and the body is more prone to disease. A recent study by the U.S. Surgeon General reported that stress can be a factor in cardiovascular disease, gastrointestinal disorders, mental illness, and even death.

There are two parts to managing stress: (1) learning to relax and (2) changing your thoughts. This book will help you incorporate into your everyday life different techniques, simple yet effective, to help you learn how to relax. You will use the power of your mind to change the thoughts that can trigger stress.

This book will inspire and instill in you an appreciation of finding a deeper beauty and meaning whenever you see flowers and plants that grow on your own windowsill or in your garden. You will enjoy using the easy-to-follow instructions and feel the empowerment that comes with the positive results and *reduction of stress!*

Follow all guidelines and instructions carefully. If a formula is found to be more powerful than desired, cut the recipe in half and work from there. People with serious medical problems such as epilepsy, schizophrenia, cancer, and heart disease, as well as pregnant women and those who are in poor health or in extremely weakened condition, should not do the baths. Keep in mind that this book is intended as an informational guide. The remedies, approaches, and techniques described within are meant to supplement rather than substitute for professional medical care or treatment. They should not be used to treat a serious ailment without prior consultation with a qualified healthcare professional.

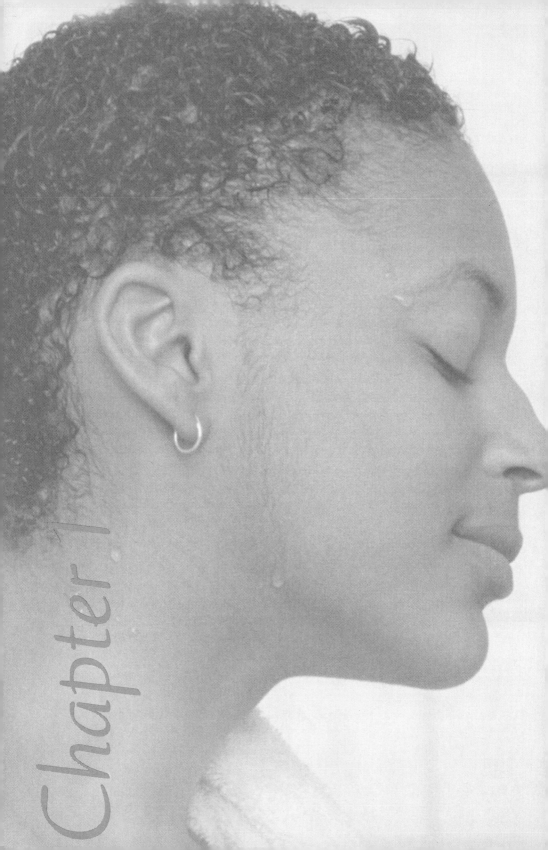

Chapter 1

the
Mind-Body-Spirit
Connection

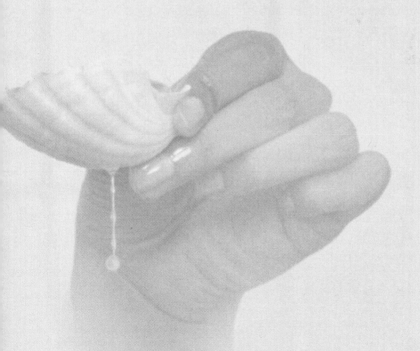

*I*s it really possible for the fragrance of an essential oil to influence our moods, our feelings, our state of mind, even our behavior? The answer is yes. Scents of aromatic oils distilled from plants are invaluable for promoting health and healing on the physical, mental, and emotional levels. Scientists today are just beginning to tap into the seemingly limitless boundaries of healing information that we can all use to attain health and longevity, but we do know that through aromatherapy the fragrances of aromatic oils can be used to heal and restore our bodies, minds, and spirits.

Fragrance researchers are discovering that odors can and do influence mood, evoke emotions, counteract stress, and reduce high blood pressure. Aromatherapy helps people feel better about themselves, improves temperament, aids relaxation, and, consequently, increases confidence, energy levels, and the ability to cope with stress. Even though we're not conscious of odors most of the time, the human nose is very sensitive, and is capable of distinguishing among hundreds of thousands of different odors, both faint and pungent.

In our daily lives, we perceive many scents that affect us — both consciously and unconsciously. For example, I eagerly anticipate visits with my 3-month-old godson, Johnathan. When I kiss him gently on his little head, I just want to breathe him in. It is a soft, warm, delicate "baby scent" that is so soothing to me. Similarly, when I visit my loving Italian mother-in-law, Maria, as soon as I enter her home the wonderful aromas of whatever is on the stove (and she is an absolutely excellent cook!) make my mouth water and fill me with the feeling that I'm being embraced.

In summer, when you go outside and the breeze smells lightly floral and then you pick up the scent of someone's barbecue, you might recall picnics and Fourth of July holidays and laughter. To this day, whenever I smell a newly opened can of paint, my memory goes way back to when I was a child and my older brother Raymond would repaint the entire apartment every December in preparation for the Christmas holidays. Despite the temporary chaos, I loved awakening in a newly painted room. Raymond always wanted to ring in the New Year with a clean slate and clean walls in the hope of new beginnings, and the smell of a freshly painted home reminds me of this.

Even in children the sense of smell is acute. They literally smell their food before hesitantly tasting it. At a gathering that I attended, mothers were telling funny stories of their children's escapades. I overheard one mom describe what happened when she went through her jewelry box as her small daughters looked on. She picked up an heirloom ring and told the 10-year-old that when she dies, this ring will be left to her. This daughter was ecstatic and realized the importance of the moment. The mother then asked her 6-year-old what she would like to have from the jewelry box to be left to her. The little girl replied, "Mommy, I would like you to spray a piece of paper with your perfume, so after you are gone, I can smell it and always remember you." My heart just about burst when I heard that! Scent is linked to many of our emotions, and we seem to take so many of them for granted.

Gaining a New Perspective

Physicians are responsible for patients as people, not just as diseased bodies. It is their obligation to be more than technicians who inform patients of what has gone wrong in their lives. It is their responsibility to seek adequate training so they may be a source of spiritual, emotional, and moral support when that is what's needed. Being able to guide patients in the right direction spiritually and psychologically can enhance the chances of a rapid and full recovery.

Why Aromatherapy Works

During an aromatherapy treatment, patients are more receptive to odors and to the treatment as a whole than they would be in most other therapeutic settings. When a person goes to his or her doctor for treatment of a physical ailment or symptoms, his or her emotions, spirit, and psyche will probably not be treated. This can be problematic, because the entire person — mind, body, and spirit — must be addressed in order for treatment to be completely successful.

With an aromatherapy treatment, a person is quickly relaxed. The therapist takes the time to develop a rapport with the client in order to help connect with him or her. Just one whiff of fragrance can have an immediate impact on the subtle energies of the body. It is possible to work on those energies that are often overlooked in the treatment of physical ailments. Essential oils should be viewed as a preventive measure to combat the negative effects of stress and as a bolster for the immune system.

As well as being very sensitive to odor, the brain is vulnerable to smells in another sense: Scents enjoy an immediate access to the brain that is denied most other remedies or drugs. There are two distinct reasons for this.

First, smell is the only sense in which the receptor nerve endings are in direct contact with the outside world; your brain extends directly into your nose! Similar to the sense of touch, smell is a primitive sense and is most likely to be loaded with instinctive associations. Second, we must consider the blood-brain barrier. The walls of the capillaries that carry blood around the brain are very selective. Although tiny nutrient and oxygen molecules can pass through the capillary walls, larger

A Pleasant Association

Many years ago I visited my Uncle Chano and Aunt Mary in Puerto Rico. Outside the house were lush, abundant gardenia bushes. The scent was intoxicating, and at night we'd sit out on the porch and enjoy the aromas from the flowers. At bedtime, they would cut gardenias for me and place them on my pillow so I would have sweet-scented dreams. To this day, gardenias are my favorite flowers, largely because I associate them with this wonderful experience.

molecules, including those found in most therapeutic drugs, cannot. Aromatherapy bypasses the barrier by going straight to the brain through the olfactory system. The essential oil itself goes no farther than the inside of the nose, but it triggers a nerve impulse, amplified along the way, that has far-reaching repercussions.

The Ancient Roots of Aromatherapy

Aromatherapy is not a new form of health therapy, despite some of the "trendiness" that currently surrounds it. Rather, aromatherapy is an ancient art of healing that has been practiced by numerous cultures in very diverse parts of the world. Even though we don't know exactly *how* aromatherapy works, we know that it *does* work in making the mind-body connection that is essential to self-healing. The ancients had more wisdom than we give them credit for.

Ancient cultures recognized the compelling power of odors on the psyche. Aromatic woods and herbs were used to drive out "evil spirits," and kyphi, an ancient Egyptian perfume, was said to "lull to sleep, allay anxieties, and brighten dreams" in a papyrus dating to around 2800 B.C. In ancient Greece, aromatic oils were often employed for their soporific, antidepressant, or aphrodisiac properties, and it was recognized that certain odors could improve mental alertness and aid concentration.

While the scents and modes of therapy sometimes differed, many cultures had strong traditions in aromatherapy since the earliest times.

Egypt

The Egyptians' everyday existence was permeated with scent. They valued its importance in everything they did, believed, and thrived on. Aromatherapy was being practiced in this country some 5,000 years ago.

Egyptians cherished bathing, and massage usually followed a bath. After a bath, the prosperous Egyptian woman would lie naked while slave girls massaged her with fragrant oils.

They also practiced contraception with herbs: Aromatic mixtures were blended and placed in the vagina to act as a spermicide. This ancient culture imported sandalwood, cinnamon, frankincense, and myrrh from faraway lands. They used scent in their religious practices, for medicinal healing, in treating physical and mental ailments, to preserve their food, and for magic.

Ancient Egyptians created perfumes by taking plant materials and soaking them in various fats and oils. They left the mixture out in the the sun for a few days, where the heat created a medicinal plant extract through a process called infusion. Plant extracts and oils were offered to the gods and goddesses in elaborate, carved vases that were abundant in their temples. Statues of their idols were anointed every morning with their highly prized oils in preparation for religious worship.

Apart from their incredible pyramids, the ancient Egyptians are most remembered for their mummies. Their beliefs dictated that the dead would still need their earthly bodies in the afterlife, so they went to great lengths to preserve the body with aromatic oils, and entombed with it jars and vials of essential oils.

The Egyptians were well aware of an aroma's ability to affect the emotions. Perfumes were formulated to uplift the spirits, dispel nervousness, encourage love, bring tranquillity, and induce aggression for the purpose of war. Each pharaoh was lucky enough to have a number of different perfumes blended for him.

The World's First Perfume?

> One of the sealed flasks discovered in the tomb of Tutankhamen was opened in 1922, and after 3,300 years it still had a perceptible odor. Analysis revealed the presence of spikenard and frankincense. Perhaps this is the only bottle of the world's first perfume!

Egyptian men and women washed often with scented floral waters. They wore cones of scented wax and fats on top of their heads to keep themselves fragrant and oiled in the intense heat of the desert. Even their jewelry released perfumed aromas, and their palaces were built of aromatic cedarwood because it is a natural insect repellent.

Cleopatra's Famous Fragrances

As queen of the Egyptian empire, Cleopatra used fragrance to allure and seduce. She demanded that the royal barge, which was made of aromatic cedarwood, be washed down with rose water and the sails soaked in fragrance. She enveloped herself and her surroundings with an abundance of perfumed oils in her quest to seduce Mark Antony.

Greece and Rome

Aromatherapy may have started in Egypt, but the Greeks developed it considerably. Aromatics were in great demand in ancient Greece and Rome. One Greek writer stated, "The best recipe for health is to apply sweet scents to the brain." These cultures had such a high regard for scent that their architectural structures were designed with rooms that opened onto their lush gardens in order to savor the fragrances.

A variety of spices, herbs, and extracts were blended in olive oil to make perfumes. The ancient Greeks and Romans even enhanced their dining experience by soaking earthenware cups and platters in scent prior to use. Doves were dipped in scented waters and then released above dinner guests; as they flew, they would weave a tapestry of scent in the air.

The Roman emperors used fragrance liberally. Caligula spent enormous sums on scented ointments, and was a great believer in the efficiency of aromatic baths to restore a body ravaged by sexual excesses. The Greeks and Romans also believed that aromatics could temper the narcotic effects of alcohol and help prevent a hangover. This led to their use of myrrh, violets, and roses in flavoring wine, and foods prepared with rose petals were always in abundance at the famous feasts and orgies.

As Roman soldiers marched into battle, they carried myrrh with them to heal their wounds. Knowledge of the healing properties of plants spread throughout the growing Roman empire. Wherever they went, they collected and planted seeds.

Asia

It seems that the ancient civilizations of India and China were practicing some form of aromatherapy during the same period as the Egyptians. It is recorded that 5,000 years ago, the Chinese living along the banks of the Yellow River were using calamus roots and mugwort leaves as hygiene aids. They also burned aromatic woods and herbs as incense in honor and tribute to their gods.

Aromatic herbs and massage were being used in China at this early period, long before the birth of Christ. Emperor Shen Nung's medical text *Herbal*, which dates back to about 2700 B.C. contains details on 365 types of plants. Emperor Huang Ti is credited with *The Yellow Emperor's Classic of Internal Medicine* (2650 B.C.). This work referred to aromatic medicines used with massage and formed the basis for acupuncture.

The oldest form of Indian medicine is known as *ayurveda*, meaning "knowledge of longevity." It has been practiced for at least 3,000 years and is still widely practiced in India today. A principal aspect of ayurveda is aromatic massage. In the early days, some essential oils were used, especially sandalwood. One of the oldest-known Indian books on plants, called *Vedas*, mentions medicinal uses for basil, cinnamon, coriander, ginger, myrrh, and sandalwood.

Builders of mosques used to mix rose water and musk into the mortar so that at noon the sun would heat it and bring out the per-

Scent and Tantra

India had an abundance of fragrant plants and flowers that were used to ensure pleasure in sexual union; tantra, the ancient Eastern practice of spiritual enlightenment that weaves spirituality and sexuality into one harmonius whole, makes use of many different scents. Indian women would comb spikenard into their long hair for the seduction of their men. In addition, part of the spiritual discipline of foreplay included a large array of tantric perfumes.

fumed aromas. Even today in India people put rose, sandalwood, frank-incense, and jasmine oil on their bodies before prayer and meditation. Jesus supposedly had his feet anointed with spikenard oil by Mary Magdalene.

The Middle East

The Persians used perfumed waters for many centuries, and the invention of distillation is credited to them. Rose water was the most popular perfumed water and the Persians exported it to China, India, and Europe. The Arabs made great advances in chemistry at this time and discovered how to make alcohol. With both alcohol and essential oils, the production of perfume without a heavy oil base became possible for the first time.

The Persian physician and scholar Avicenna (A.D. 980–1037) refined the process of distillation, and then exported the process to China, Europe, and India to be used for medicinal and culinary purposes. Perfumes were formulated using roses, lilies, narcissi, and violets. In his book *The Canon of Medicine,* Avicenna mentions the use of many essential oils, including chamomile, cinnamon, peppermint, and dill. This particular book was used as a standard reference by many medieval schools until the middle of the 16th century.

American Indians

The Cherokee believe that all illness, whether acute or chronic, begins at the spiritual level. If you think about the last time your child developed an ear infection, for example, you may have noticed there was a change in his "spirit" or energy several days before the ear actually began to ache. You may also remember something occurring that may have been traumatic, however slight, to the child. That event can weaken the spirit temporarily, and that, in turn, can weaken the immune system.

Native Americans have true harmony and reverence for the earth. They use plants for various practical purposes but also for ritualistic spiritual practices. They are one with Mother Earth and believe in maintaining a balance with the spiritual and physical aspects of nature.

The Cherokee, as well as the Omaha and Ponca tribes, burned wild sage to purify an area of negative energies and evil spirits. Similarly, if a tribal law was broken, the offender would have to bathe with the sage plant. The herb also was used in many of their ceremonies. The chewed root of this plant was placed on clothing to attract good luck, protection, and love and to ensure good hunting for the Winnebago tribe. They would allow the wind to bring the scent of sage to whatever it was that they wished to attract. It was combined with visualization of the desired wish or outcome.

Among some tribes, dried sweetgrass was braided and the end was ignited in a ceremony to invoke the presence of good spirits. Sweetgrass, which smells like vanilla when burned, was also added to mixtures that were smoked during pipe ceremonies to summon good powers. The root of the yellow evening primrose was rubbed onto a hunter's clothes, moccasins, and body; the scent attracted deer, yet repelled snakes.

The ancient Hawaiians were known for their skill at massage and their use of scented oils. The grated meat of coconut was placed with other plant materials in dried gourds in the hot sun. Water was poured over the mixture, and the heat of the sun caused the plants' essential oils to separate and float on the water. It would then be strained and used as a fragrant skin softener and as protection against countless hours of swimming in the ocean.

Ancient Tricks

Sage baths are used for assisting a person to gain true wisdom. Use the leaf or powdered form of the herb along with 3 drops of sage essential oil. Bathe in it on a Thursday at sunrise. While in the bath, review the events of the week and your responses or reactions to those events. Immerse yourself nine times by sitting up out of the water and then sliding back under again. Remain in the bath at least 9 minutes. This mystical plant will aid in the destruction of illusion, which will leave you in a state of clarity and wisdom!

Aromatherapy in the 20th Century

Aromatherapy had fallen into disfavor in the 18th century among the cultures of the developed world as strides were made in treating disease with allopathic medicine. Only recently, as the public clamors for information on all-natural, side-effect-less treatments, has aromatherapy come close to widespread acceptance, due to the work of several pioneering scientists.

Perfumer and chemist René-Maurice Gattefosse examined the surprisingly positive healing effects of essential oils. While working in Grasse, France, he coined the term "aromatherapy," including it in a book he published in 1937 on the antimicrobial effects of essential oils. Gattefosse is credited with the discovery of the therapeutic benefits of lavender oil. In an excerpt from his book *Aromathérapie* he writes, "External application of small quantities of essential oils rapidly stops the spread of gangrenous sores. In my personal experience after a laboratory explosion covered me with burning substances which I extinguished by rolling on my grassy lawn, my hands were covered with a rapidly changing gas gangrene. Just one rinse with lavender oil stopped the gastrification of the tissues. The treatment was followed by profuse sweating and healing began the next day."

After his research, lavender oil was used for everything, including open wounds in which all tissue was gone and the bones were revealed. This oil is an anti-inflammatory and the healing agent for burns, open wounds, and sores. It is also a powerful antiseptic.

At the same time in Australia, the benefits of tea tree oil were discovered. During the Second World War, army surgeon Dr. Jean Valnet had been so greatly influenced by the research of Gattefosse that he used essential oils as antiseptics in the treatment of battle wounds. After the war, he continued using the oils in his capacity as a doctor, and in 1964 published a comprehensive work also entitled Aromathérapie, which earned him international recognition.

Soon after, Valnet began teaching other doctors about the healing benefits of essential oils. Due to his pioneering research, there are currently at least four establishments in France where medical doctors can learn aromatherapy. Some 1,500 practitioners now prescribe essential oils. Let us hope that doctors all over the world will follow this example.

Between 1920 and 1930, Italian scientists and doctors Giovanni Gatti and Renato Cayola conducted experiments dealing with the psychological effects of essential oils. They published an article in 1922 entitled "The Action of Essences on the Nervous System" that discussed the effects of essential oils on this important body system, including their stimulating and calming properties. Gatti and Cayola measured blood pressure, pulse rate, blood circulation, and breathing frequency of patients who were exposed to the scent of an essential oil. They also observed the positive capacity of essential oils in destroying bacteria. Always ahead of their time, the doctors recommended jasmine and lemon essential oils for the treatment of depression and anxiety.

Madame Marguerite Maury introduced aromatherapy into Britain in the 1950s. She diluted essential oils in a carrier oil for use in massage. Maury was instrumental in teaching her techniques to beauty therapists, and she wrote *The Secret of Life and Youth,* an in-depth research report on rejuvenation through the use of essential oils and massage. She recognized the value of ancient teachings, so she wrote of the various philosophies practiced by Hindu, Chinese, and Tibetan medicine. Madame Maury, who was born in 1885, practiced and taught aromatherapy until her death in 1964.

Several doctors and researchers have made valuable contributions to aromatherapy during the last 20 to 30 years, especially Professor Paolo Rovesti, of Milan University in Italy. Rovesti asserted, "Aromatherapy . . . is not just another medicine, a heretical and unofficial one. On the contrary, it has come through experimental method to occupy its rightful place among the most effective remedies in therapeutic use."

Contemporary Theories

Smell is one of the most important and basic senses. The scientific term for this sense is olfaction and the system by which we smell is known as the olfactory system. Surprisingly, olfactory nerve cells are the only types of nerve cells in the body that can be replaced if damaged.

How Odors Are Detected

The cells that are part of the olfactory nerves rest on layers of mucus-covered tissue. This tissue covers nasal bones called conchae. We detect smells by breathing or sniffing air that carries odors. Odors come from molecules of gas that are made up of many different substances. These molecules stimulate receptor cells deep inside the nose, which then send the impulses created by the odor along the olfactory nerves.

The olfactory nerves then carry the impulses to a part of the brain called the olfactory lobe or olfactory bulb. From the olfactory lobe, the nerve impulses travel to the forebrain, the front part of the cerebrum. Here, the brain translates the nerve impulses it has received into information about the odor.

Scientists do not know exactly how different smells are distinguished. One explanation is that molecules of certain odors become more quickly and more strongly attached to the mucus at a particular place on the conchae than do other molecules. Those molecules will always stimulate the same receptor cells on the conchae, thus forming the basis of scent recognition.

Scent and Recognition

Napoleon told Josephine not to bathe during the two weeks that would pass before they met, so he could enjoy her in all her natural aromas. Napoleon and Josephine also adored violets, and her violet-scented perfume was her trademark. When Josephine died, in 1814, Napoleon planted violets at her grave. Just before his exile he made a pilgrimage to her grave site, picked some of the violets, and enclosed them in a locket, which he wore until the end of his life.

How the Brain Interprets Scent

Odors do affect us, even if we do not consciously perceive them. Sometimes people find the concept of therapeutic aromas difficult to accept. This is not surprising because our conscious mind is frequently unaware of the presence of odors.

There are several ways in which olfaction and memory are related. Most importantly, we must recognize that two olfactory nerve tracts run right into the limbic system, the area of the brain that contains the main centers for both memory and olfaction. Because of this, you can experience a variety of specific feelings, emotions, memories, and moods — such as relaxation, exhilaration, sensuality, and happiness — when stimulated by a particular scent. Scents can evoke an immediate and strong response.

Inhaled essential oils reach the body through the lungs and bloodstream or through the nose, then progress to the limbic system. Here the essences trigger a release of hormones and neurochemicals to create mental and emotional effects. Just taking a sniff of a specific scent can recall memories. If certain scents bring up memories of pain and suffering, you might relive those emotions when exposed to that aroma. You can either interpret the reaction as a helpful way to release this kind of pain, or you might choose to avoid this particular scent. A smell can be incredibly powerful because it can trigger all types of memories and emotions before we have time to "edit" them.

Females score higher than males in tests that measure sensitivity to odors, regardless of age group. Women in general have a stronger sense of smell, which is cyclical, as it changes during menstruation and is influenced by hormones. During the first half of the menstrual cycle,

Using Smell Every Day

We employ our sense of smell daily to check out and then enjoy the food we eat. Picture yourself at a restaurant. Your meal has arrived and the first forkful passes by your nose before it gets to your mouth. If something smells awkward or "funny," you might not even allow yourself to taste it. But when you walk by a bakery, doesn't the smell wafting out stimulate your taste buds? Much of the taste of food depends on its smell. If you have a cold and a stuffed-up nose and can't smell what you are eating, chances are you also can barely taste your food. We derive pleasure simply from the odor of our favorite foods cooking, just as we enjoy the fragrance of perfume or flowers.

when estrogen levels are high, a woman's sense of smell is heightened. If a woman's ovaries are removed, however, she will lose the ability to detect "musk" scents; this is because musk scents are linked with attraction and procreation, an ability that is lost when the ovaries are removed. But once given artificial estrogen, her recognition of this type of scent is then restored.

Aromatherapy as a Way of Life

Fragrance is a form of nonverbal communication in which messages are exchanged between people, carrying fully developed ideas and emotions. Fragrance companies have discovered that nationality or culture also influences the perception of fragrances. For example, Germans like piney scents, the French prefer flowery aromas, the Japanese favor more delicate fragrances, and South Americans want stronger scents. Floor-cleaning products in Venezuela contain 10 times as much pine scent as do those sold in the United States!

Because of the millions of dollars for research paid by the fragrance industry, the effect of inhaled essential oils on the brain is well documented. This process of scent recognition has a profound impact on the endocrine and nervous systems, the emotions, memory, and more. That is why the inhalation of essential oils is so effective in the treatment of emotional and mental imbalances; it treats the person as a "whole," rather than treating just a couple of parts. And aromatherapy has obvious benefits for the respiratory system in treating diseases such as asthma, emphysema, bronchitis, tuberculosis, pneumonia, and the common cold.

The greatest attraction of aromatherapy is that the treatments smell good, and things that smell good always make us feel better! Aromatherapy is a way of life, an opportunity to take your own well-being in hand. Essential oils influence our consciousness, reconnect us with plants and the phenomenon of life. Scent allows us to breathe in and then release our emotions of the day. Scent helps to revitalize and refresh our spirits. Most importantly in this modern world, aromatherapy allows us to let go of stress, as it encourages us to slow our pace and breathe in life itself.

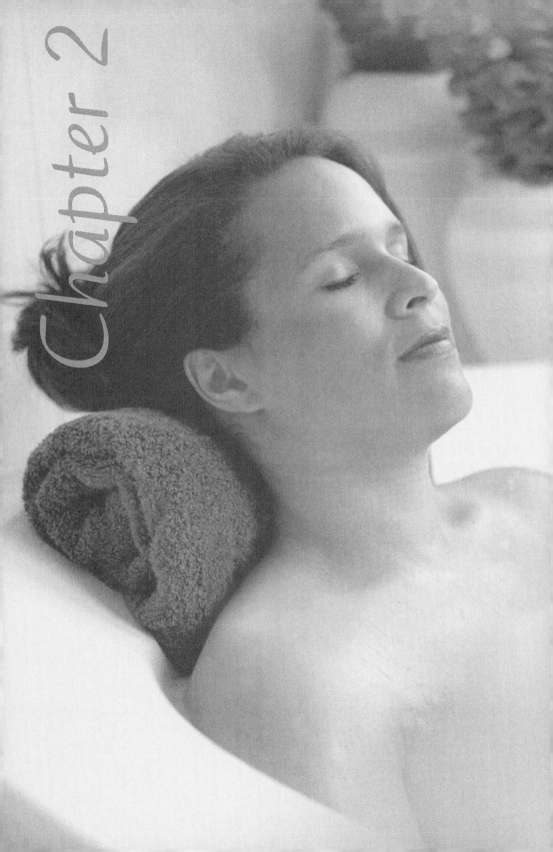

Chapter 2

simple

Visualization

Techniques

for

Self-Discovery

*T*here has always been a mystique surrounding hypnosis, a sense of the unknown that is both intriguing and frightening. But there is nothing to fear from this approach, which works with your subconscious mind. You can perform some simple exercises that will help you develop a cooperative relationship with your inner self, a connection that is likely to lead to healing and greater fulfillment.

What Is Hypnosis?

The term "hypnosis" comes from the Greek root word *hypnos,* meaning "sleep." It refers to a state of consciousness that allows a variety of mental and behavioral responses to be stimulated. As a result of suggestions made to the unconscious, even memory patterns and the awareness of self may be changed.

Despite the misconceptions, hypnosis is not really mysterious. Once learned, it is a tool that allows a person to use more of his or her mind and to use it more dynamically and effectively. Hypnosis is a restful receptivity with increased perception; it is a state of deep relaxation that quiets the body and opens the mind. With its defenses down, the mind is especially open to suggestion, the type of which is determined by a person's goals and ideals and the reason for using hypnosis.

Hypnosis is also a method of relaxing the physical body and utilizing another level of awareness. This level of awareness, called alpha, refers to a state of electrical activity in the brain.

Using Hypnosis to Heal Yourself

Your subconscious mind is your secret garden where the thoughts you plant grow to become your reality. This garden is far more fertile than you may realize.

Like a gardener, you choose the "thought seeds" you want to plant. Mental techniques combined with the power of aromatherapy enable you to care for and nourish those thought seeds, helping them grow and bear fruit; you directly create a physical reality that manifests whatever you desire. The seeds that grow will empower you with positive thinking, happiness, confidence, forgiveness, love, and acceptance and will create balance and spiritual abundance. It is your responsibility to create the harmony for yourself in this lifetime.

I will show you how to take more control of your own mind and gear it toward accomplishing your objectives with the self-hypnosis techniques of guided imagery, meditation, visualization, and affirmation. You will develop mental strength and become more connected to your spiritual core. You can build your mind and remodel your life the way you want it to be. You'll be able to change the way you respond to people and situations you formerly had problems with. While aromatherapy won't transform an unreasonable boss, you will no longer allow your energy to be depleted from anger and frustration. You cannot change the demeanor of someone you don't like, but you *can* change how it affects you.

Self-Hypnosis Terms and Techniques

With my aromatherapy blends and the addition of any of these four techniques, you will achieve a deep inner cleansing and clearing that will help to nourish and fortify your body, mind, and spirit. As you break down negative programming, you will see fast and dramatic changes in your life. Great empowerment develops and continues to grow as you release what blocks your path to achieving your full potential.

Guided imagery. A method of directing the course of mental images.

Meditation. The act of thinking deeply, utilizing concentration in its highest form.

Visualization. A method of forming a mental image of something not present to the sight.

Affirmation. Using words to verbalize thoughts into a positive declaration, a statement of truth that one aspires to absorb into one's life.

Progressive Relaxation

A progressive relaxation exercise focuses on the tensing and relaxing of different muscle groups for the purpose of releasing stress. This type of exercise can be done before going to sleep, before going out for the day, or even before your visualization exercises. It will help rid you of anxiety, allowing for deep relaxation. You will experience an increased awareness of internal functions and an increased receptivity of the senses. Once your body is relaxed, you will find it easier for your mind to focus.

Progressive Relaxation Exercise

1. Find a quiet place. Loosen your clothing and either sit or lie down.

2. Begin breathing. Most of the time we breathe from the upper lobes of the lungs, which have a much smaller capacity than do our lower lungs. Breathe, instead, with your diaphragm. Inhale slowly to the count of 8. Expand your belly so that the bottom parts of the lungs can take in air. Hold your breath for a count of 4, then exhale slowly for a count of 8.

3. Wait for a count of 4, then repeat the entire breathing process. By the second sequence you'll already find yourself beginning to relax. Do this throughout the remainder of the relaxation session.

4. Tense your facial and scalp muscles. Hold for a count of 4, then release them. Feel the tension flow out.

5. Move your head and neck forward, backward, and side to side, tensing the muscles as you move. Hold the tension for a count of 4, then relax slowly. Take in the relaxation, allowing the stress to spill away.

6. Tense your shoulder muscles. Hold for a count of 4, then release. The tension continues to evaporate. Tense your arm muscles, then your hands, and hold for a count of 4. Release the tension. Feel the stress disappear.

7. Repeat this tensing and releasing through the rest of your body, from the chest, to the stomach, to the hips, to the buttocks, to the thighs, and then the calves, feet, and toes. When you finally release your toe muscles, you should feel all of the built-up stress pour out through your feet.

8. You will now feel totally relaxed. Lie there for a few minutes and allow yourself to drift in the blissful feeling of pure relaxation you have created.

Guided Imagery

Through this practice, you attempt to stimulate changes in body functions usually considered inaccessible to conscious influence. Doctors are still trying to explain how guided imagery might play a role in alleviating pain and discomfort. Many researchers think the "relaxation response" is a key factor.

In directing the course of mental images, you experience a guided journey into the creative center of the mind. Here you can manifest your hopes and dreams, and put into motion the energy necessary to achieve them.

The Benefits

Guided imagery is a form of self-hypnosis that scientific research has associated with positive stimulation of the immune system and enhanced feelings of well-being and self-empowerment. This technique helps heal emotional and physical upsets by getting in touch with your healing source of energy and strength. Many counselors, psychologists, therapists, ministers, nurses, and other mental health professionals practice and use relaxation and guided imagery techniques in their training.

Basically, guided imagery consists of using all of your concentration to build a picture of yourself as healthy. A simple way is to imagine wellness right where there is discomfort or sickness. Suppose you have a sprained ankle or an internal organ that needs healing. All you do is imagine that part as already healed and keep concentrating on that image, despite what the present condition is. This image will serve as a guide to the body's "consciousness" and help it to bring about the healed condition more rapidly.

In quite a few cultures, healers had very good results when the imagined "picture" was combined with a healing suggestion phrased in the form of rhyming chants. Sometimes the chants would be directed to the gods and spirits, but they were still absorbed and remembered by the sick person's subconscious. You can make up your own form of "self-suggestion" that reaches deep into your subconscious and sticks. For example, tell yourself, "The power of life is flowing in me and through me. My body is healing perfectly." Or try saying, "With strong intent and powerful feeling, my body receives a perfect healing." Keep your conscious mind busy with the expectation of the best, and your subconscious mind will help your body faithfully reproduce your habitual thinking.

Most diseases are a result of negative thinking, feeling, and acting. Research suggests that by dwelling on negative emotions, we trigger physical reactions that use up our vital energies and lower the body's resistance to all types of diseases, whether they are physical, mental, or spiritual.

For instance, if we hold hatred for someone in our hearts, we will pollute our consciousness with that hatred. You will become angry with and mean to others. People pick up on this negative energy and steer clear of you. Blocking joy and happiness from entering your life wears down your immune system. You'll miss out on the beauty of all life that surrounds you, and wind up attracting more hatred and anger to your life. In time the hatred and resentment will overwhelm the heart. When you blow up at someone or something, you are putting tremendous demands on your heart, making it pump harder and less efficiently. If you are prone to fits of losing your temper, then you risk immediate and harmful changes to your heart. The secret is to cool it before your anger boils over. (See pages 126–131 for more information on releasing anger.)

Our consciousness is like a container that continues to hold whatever we decide to put into it, both life-promoting and life-diminishing impulses. We can bring into our consciousness and remove from it whatever we choose. Guided imagery is one step toward bringing positive perceptions into our consciousness by influencing the underlying part — the unconscious.

If we think back over our youth and reflect on our predominant personality traits, then we can begin to have some insight into some of our characteristics. If someone repeatedly told you that you weren't as smart or attractive as someone else, or that you were clumsy, these negative thoughts became ingrained in your being; you began to believe what you heard. But we can learn how to remove these patterns that have resulted in unhappiness and misunderstanding. By retraining our thoughts and emotions, the light of our souls will again be able to shine bright.

Guided imagery is a creative technique that uses your active mind to create a picture. That picture is used for the basis of altering your current condition, transforming a negative state into a positive one. It is truly a reflection of that old adage, "Mind over matter."

Simple Guided Imagery Exercise

1. Select a cool room for this exercise; be sure it is free of distractions like phones or TVs. Open a window slightly and feel the breeze.

2. Sit in a recliner or lie flat on your back on a bed or on the floor on a mat or comforter.

3. Close your eyes and take a deep breath. Hold the breath for a moment, then release. Repeat. Breathe in while visualizing the word "relax." Breathe out while visualizing the word "release."

4. Now imagine a bright orange ball of energy right above your head. It is pulsating with vibrancy and strength. Visualize a heavy electrical cord coming out of the ball, dangling toward you.

5. Imagine yourself plugging the cord into a socket in your right temple. Keep the image in your mind for at least 1 full minute. Feel the energy surging through your brain and into your body.

6. If necessary, keep visualizing the scene for a longer period. You can do this for as long as it takes for you to experience a revitalizing feeling. Try this exercise whenever you need to reenergize at work, or before going out for the evening after a hectic, tiring day.

Meditation

Meditation is excellent for everyone, especially those people who are seeking to heal their physical ailments, feel energized and more optimistic, and improve their lifestyle. It is exercise for the mind that has incredible healing powers.

Four thousand years ago the Tibetans recognized the mind-body connection, recording their observations in *The Yellow Emperor's Book of Internal Medicine*. But it wasn't until recently that scientists realized its potential. When Herbert Benson, M.D., first published *The Relaxation Response,* the evidence of this connection was overwhelming. His intricate studies showed the positive effect meditation has on lowering blood pressure. Now, Harvard Medical School is home to the Benson Mind-Body Medical Institute, which uses meditation as a treatment for serious illness, as well as high blood pressure.

The Benefits

When you meditate, you concentrate deeply and experience continuous contemplation. Meditation encourages and deepens wisdom. With this process, you can enter directly through the mind and heal the heart. Both visualization and meditation have become important tools in treating disorders such as cancer, heart problems, and diseases of the immune system. I was in awe at a lecture I attended that featured Dr. Bernie Siegel, whose books stress the healing powers of the mind. He told us that there are two ways to communicate these messages from the mind to the body: One is through the emotions. Dr. Siegel says that he tells patients, "If you want to die, stay depressed. If you want to live, then love and laugh." Positive emotions attained through meditation like love, acceptance, and forgiveness revitalize the immune system and contribute to overall well-being.

Through meditation you can attain a state of awareness where the mind is free of thoughts and worries. Consciousness is the awareness of your being — it is the recognition of your "self" within yourself. Your outside "self" is your body, your inside "self" is an awareness, something you cannot see but you know is there. The mind and consciousness operate together; consciousness uses the mind as its tool for producing thoughts. Meditation is one of the ways in which a state of peace can be experienced by stilling your body and letting go of the mind. It improves physical and mental health and helps a person deal with stress.

Meditation relies on the body's ability to switch to an alpha (resting) or theta (relaxing) brain-wave state, during which the brain's rhythm slows down, and endorphins, the body's natural painkiller, are released. Studies have shown that during meditation the heart rate is lowered, blood pressure decreases, and breathing slows down; you decrease the consumption of oxygen by as much as 20 percent. Blood lactates, a high level of which are associated with anxiety attacks, decrease. Stress on the heart and other organs is reduced. Meditation relieves fatigue, helps you to cope with your anxieties, reduces stress, and helps you sleep better. It helps to increase attention span and can aid the development of patience and composure. In turn, you become more alert and focused, and your body's hidden defenses against stress and stress-triggered illnesses are released.

Like the other methods suggested here, meditation takes a holistic approach, involving both the mind and the body. By turning your attention inward you can become familiar with your deepest thoughts and feelings. By being more in touch with yourself, you have greater control over your outlook and, therefore, the quality of your own life. As you develop a new kind of awareness, sensations become more vivid, your ability to concentrate increases, and creativity is enhanced. You will learn to look inside, to look to yourself rather than other people for approval. You will trust in your own judgments to help you cope with everyday pressures and, in this way, will increase your mental and physical well-being.

With meditation, you can experience peace by becoming the master of your own mind. It takes a conscious desire and effort to calm the mind and look inward at yourself rather than outward at the world. You learn to draw on your inner resources for inspiration and direction. Many athletes achieve peak performance by practicing meditative visualization. When you use your concentration to visualize yourself already accomplishing a goal, your mind and body assume you have done so.

Likewise, certain thoughts produce related emotions. If you think sad thoughts, you experience unhappiness. If you think fearful thoughts, you experience anxiety. If you think joyful thoughts, you experience happiness. Express more love, light, truth, and beauty and you will become one of the happiest people in the world.

With this state of heightened consciousness, you experience an inner way of traveling that carries you through the scenery of your own mind: a journey made by thoughts or feelings, by the constant play of your own inner experience. It is a journey that embraces daily life and the magical flights of imagination that take us where we need to be. It is the journey of being alive that teaches us a way, a path to take. Meditation helps you attain the transforming attitudes necessary to rise above self-limiting habits and develops life-promoting ones. It is from that joy of simply being — in a state of stillness — that healing arises in the mind and brings us home to the heart of understanding. You can begin realizing your highest potential. Make a true effort to go within, and you will find there all that you longed for: happiness.

Simple Meditation Exercise

1. Pick a comfortable room that is free of distractions. Be sure it is warm enough; your blood pressure will drop a little during this exercise. Darken the room. Light a candle and place it in front of you.

2. Gaze at the candle for several seconds. Close your eyes.

3. Visualize the flame glowing on the back of your forehead as you "look" at the darkness behind your eyes. The image may be momentary, glowing and then fading. Try to see the details of the candle. Can you see the formation of the melting wax? Can you see the different colors within the flame? Can you hold on to the complete image in front of you?

4. You might find that you want to open your eyes to grasp certain details, but try to keep your eyes closed. It takes practice to acquire this skill, but you will improve your ability to retain the mental picture more easily. Continue to practice this exercise until you feel comfortable with it and your level of focus.

5. Try this exercise with other objects such as a flower or a piece of fruit. You can also create your own colorful scene within your mind. Focus on the details, and keep the image in your mind without becoming distracted by outside elements.

Visualization

Visualization starts in the imagination, forming a mental picture of what you desire to create in the universe. The more clearly you form the mental picture in your mind, the more accurately it will be produced as a physical fact. Using visualization, you can restore yourself by building strong pictures in your mind of the healing taking place and the outcome that you seek. Work on strongly believing that these mind pictures are real.

The Benefits

Visualization has become an important tool in treating cancer, heart problems, and diseases of the immune system, and for good reason. In a calm, relaxed state, when you consciously put forth a clear request, whatever you hope, dream, and desire will come to you. You are using your imagination to create what you want to manifest in your life.

What if you want to attract the ideal partner in love? Begin now to impress your subconscious mind with the personal qualities and characteristics that you would desire in that person. Sit in a chair, close your eyes, let go, and relax the body. Take some deep, long breaths and allow yourself to become very quiet — passive yet receptive. Talk to your subconscious mind. Say to it, "I am now attracting a man/woman into my life who is honest, kind, sincere, faithful, peaceful, considerate, romantic, happy, and prosperous. These qualities that I admire are sinking deep down into my subconscious mind now. As I concentrate on these characteristics, they become a part of me and are deeply rooted subconsciously. I will attract that which I feel to be true in my subconscious mind and beliefs. There is mutual love, freedom, and respect."

This is not to say that you will necessarily attract the most physically gorgeous or absolutely perfect partner, but by impregnating your subconscious mind with positive thoughts, you will be able to attract a mate possessing the inner qualities and characteristics you have contemplated. I practiced this meditation technique with prayer and I am now so happily married to a wonderful man that my endorphins are constantly stimulated; I feel a blissful joy like no other. Be receptive to this gift of love that you have given to your subconscious mind. You can attract love by creating an atmosphere of love in your life. Your attitude determines whom you attract into your world.

Visualization is the art of creating mental images. Many people use creative visualization without being aware of it. We might envision the proceedings of a meeting at work, or see ourselves outside, participating in our daily 5 o'clock jog. Perhaps you are looking forward to your vacation, picturing yourself relaxing on a tropical beach or going for an exhilarating run down a perfect white ski slope. Each of these scenarios will likely bring up a corresponding emotion; in the case of the meeting you might feel nervous, while you'll probably feel joyful and eager at the thought of a ski trip. The key is to visualize yourself as successful in these scenes, and a positive result is sure to follow.

Because of our own deep-seated negative ideas about life, we have automatically and unconsciously expected and imagined the worst is yet to come; limitation, difficulties, and problems are often what we expect. Through events or interactions with certain types of people and situations, we have developed deep grooves of mental and emotional responses that are automatic. Many people are not aware that they are programmed to respond to situations from a pattern that they set up years ago. For example, if as a child you fell down the stairs and badly hurt yourself, you have ingrained in your memory the pain, the trauma, the fear. Now every time you take the stairs, you might hold tightly onto the banister and walk carefully without even realizing it. Your focus gets stuck in a negative way of thinking, and as a result, that is what you create for yourself and bring to your life.

By tapping into and using your thoughts in a more conscious way, you use your imagination to create and attract what your heart desires. You can have more loving and satisfying relationships, rewarding work, more enthusiasm and enjoyment of every day. Stress reduction, increased health, wealth, a love of life, a love for other people, and a heightened appreciation for each and every day of your life can be attained — if you believe in yourself and want to accomplish it!

Everyone has the ability to use his or her imagination to create a mental picture. These pictures are usually accompanied by a strong sense or feeling. You must concentrate fully on that image or feeling of what you want to manifest in your life. Open up all of your senses to it — bring in the sensations of taste, smell, sound, and sight. Feel free to add detail and embellishment. As an exercise, create a scene or vacation place that you've been to that was a positive experience for you. Close your eyes, see the mountaintop, stream, or other special location. For me it's a beach in the Caribbean. I feel the warm sand under my feet, smell the salty ocean, and hear seagulls cry and waves crash on the shoreline. I can see and hear the palm trees rustling in the breeze, I can feel the sun on my skin, I can taste the salty, damp air. This is what I mean by opening up all your senses to the experience.

By visualizing the desired outcome as already accomplished or achieved, tap into what that joyful sensation feels like in your heart and soul. Bring it into every fiber of your being; feel it radiate throughout your body. There will be a shift in your consciousness. You will be able to break down internal barriers that have kept you from happiness and sabotaged your performance — even before you start on your task or desire.

Learn to create wonderful moments in your life, first with thoughts that set the necessary energy into motion to bring completion. When you begin to trust in the results this can bring, you can accomplish amazing things that just start with a thought. Attract the good that the universe has to offer.

Simple Visualization Exercise

1. Select a nice, warm room that is free of distractions. Lie or sit down on a comfortable piece of furniture or carpet. You are now ready to take a mental "vacation."

2. Focus on the sound of your breath moving in and out. Feel the breath as it enters and exits your body. Do this for about 1 minute.

3. Visualize yourself on an isolated mountaintop, looking out over the peaceful countryside. There is a cool, shaded stream running below. If you'd rather visualize a spot that is your special, quiet place, do so. See, feel, and taste your surroundings. Stay there for a couple of minutes, taking in the entire experience. Try not to let your mind wander from the scene.

4. When you are ready, bring yourself back to the room. You will be amazed at how much more relaxed and refreshed you will feel.

Affirmation

An affirmation is a positive thought or idea that you consciously focus on in order to produce a desired result. It is a simple technique that can heal and transform your innermost thoughts and beliefs. In a language it can hear and understand, affirmations reach the subconscious. You can say them to yourself silently, but I prefer to say them aloud. They can be powerful and effective to give you a more positive, creative outlook and help you achieve specific goals. Words have immeasurable power, especially when we speak them with concentration. They are carried into the subconscious to change us on different levels of the mind, over which most of us have little conscious control. Remember: *You are what you think.*

The Benefits

You can use affirmations to shape your inner and outer reality. Your outer reality is a direct reflection of your thoughts and beliefs. When you change your thoughts, you change your reality. Because your thoughts are manifested through the written and spoken word, when you create affirmations for yourself, you should write them down, read them silently, then read them out loud. Choose to bring more love, happiness, balance, creativity, and success into your life. Here are some examples of affirmations:

~ I love and accept myself just the way I am.
~ The more I love myself, the more I love others.
~ My life is filled with abundance.
~ I choose happiness today.
~ I choose success today.
~ I choose peace today.
~ Every day in every way I am getting better and better.

After using affirmations for a time, you will experience a calmness, confidence, and decreased fear. The effect will be subtle but noticeable to you. Whenever you feel doubt or anxiety, just recite your affirmation and you will experience a state of peace and serenity. In doing this, you are programming your subconscious to believe that you will succeed in what you are affirming. The new belief will lead to the behavior that will create the outcome you want.

Take charge of your life by being aware and assuming control of your thoughts. It has been estimated that success may be as much as 98 percent mental preparation and only 2 percent outer action. The more you do your affirmations, the more rapid and powerful the healing will be. If you don't believe affirmations can work, think again: Muhammad Ali tapped into not only his natural talent, but also the power of affirmations when he was an unknown fighter named Cassius Clay. Ten years later he was hailed as the greatest boxer of all time.

Creating Affirmations

Pick an area of your life that needs healing, whether it is a relationship, your health, your job, your financial situation, your self-image, or your goals. If you have old anger that needs to be released, now is the time to create an affirmation. Decide what you want to occur in that part of your life.

When creating affirmations:

1. Write them in the present tense, as if the experience were happening in this moment. Write "I am peaceful" rather than "I will become peaceful."

2. State your affirmation positively. When you say "I am not angry," the subconscious mind screens out the word "not" and only hears "angry." Rephrase the affirmation to state directly what you want: "I now release my resentment." Experience the difference between the way these two sample statements make you feel.

3. Repeat your affirmation each day. Write it down, then read it, then say it out loud. Repetition is important; it impresses the thought pattern on your mind and reprograms your "bio-computer" to transform your previously held beliefs.

When reciting your affirmations:

1. Repeat them loudly at first to command the full attention of your conscious mind.
2. Repeat them quietly to absorb more deeply the meaning of the words.
3. Now speak them in a whisper, carrying their meaning down into the subconscious.
4. Repeat them again silently to deepen your absorption of them at the subconscious level.

At every level, repeat the affirmation several times, absorbing ever more deeply their full meaning. You can strengthen and later reflect on your awareness of any quality you want to develop. The more you use affirmations, the more rapid and powerful the healing will be. The words become a living presence in your awareness; you will "become" the words. If you repeat "I am peace," you will become peaceful. When you say "I am love," you will feel loving and become loved. Over time, your mental and emotional outlook will noticeably improve.

You have a choice to keep the beliefs that support you and release those that cause you pain. As you become more definite about your

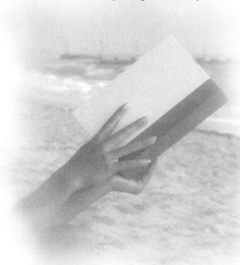

dreams and desires, they become definite about you, by turning the great energy of your thinking on realizations of plenty, whether it be health, wealth, or joy. Change your inner reality with the words you write and speak. Suggestion is accepted by the uncritical mind. What follows, then, is harmony and enlightenment.

Thoughts create reality!

Simple Affirmation Exercise for Success and Prosperity

1. To invite success and prosperity into your life, try this technique. First, set your goals in writing by making a list of the good that you want to experience in your life. Try using a small journal just for this purpose, and be sure you have privacy while doing it. Some of my favorite affirmations are, "God is now the source of my supply and my unlimited abundance," "I trust in the Universal Spirit of prosperity to provide richly for me now," "I have a constant flow of joy in my life," "Divine love is now working through me to adjust all the details of my life," and "I am guided and filled with the spirit of divine wisdom and love, and I am led to my highest good." You can use one or more affirmations on a daily basis. Be sure you are definite in your wording about success and prosperity; this is the only way for success and prosperity to be definite about *you.*

2. Read your affirmations out loud with conviction. Feel the words in your heart. Spend at least 5 minutes reciting your affirmations. Concentrate on the words and the feeling they produce; do not allow yourself to become distracted by outside interruptions.

3. You can also cut out pictures from magazines and newspapers, then glue them into your journal. These can help you visualize the success and prosperity you desire for yourself.

4. Pay close attention to the words and phrases you use during the course of a day. This is particularly important when you are discussing an area of your life that you are having some difficulty in. Listen for phrases like "I can't," "I always," and "I never," as well as other self-limiting words. These will sabotage your progress. Pick out the most negative statement you repeatedly make about yourself, and change it into a positive affirmation. Use your imagination, emotions, and concentration on this statement for an entire month and you will see improvement.

5. Recite your affirmations daily, saying them with confidence and conviction. You will open your mind to receive the abundance that is awaiting you.

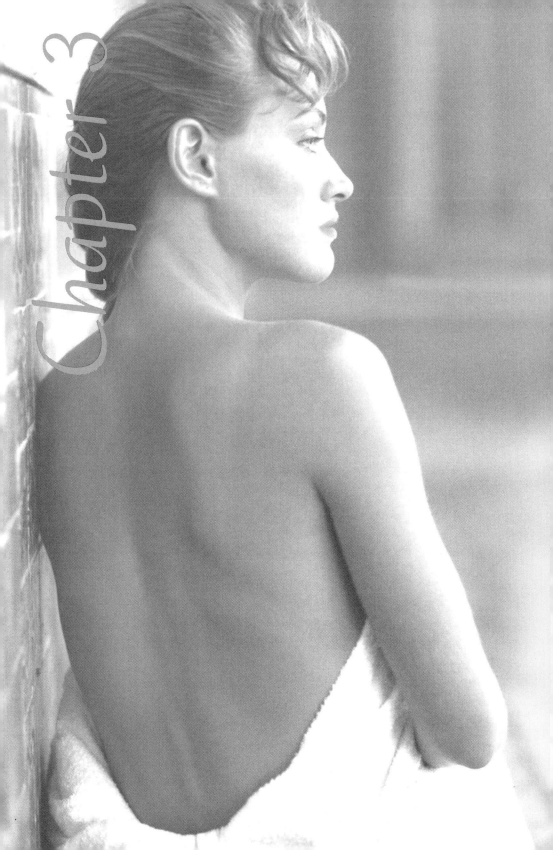

Chapter 3

Creating Healing Aromatherapy Baths

When you add essential oils to your bathwater, you will eagerly anticipate the pleasurable experience before you even place one foot in the tub! The bath holds essences that will take you to another time. Totally experiencing the power and magic of an essential oil bath is like listening to a particular piece of music that you have never heard before and being transported to a wonderful place you've never been.

Using Essential Oils

The bath became seductive and irresistible to me once I started using the different oils and beautiful extracts. You'll want to take a healing bath every day once you start adding these fragrant essential oils to your bathwater!

Essential oils give herbs, spices, fruits, and flowers their specific scent, aroma, and flavor. Each oil has individual benefits to which the mind, the body, and the spirit respond. Almost everybody — it doesn't matter what age — benefits from the use of essential oils. Pure plant oils can improve your state of mind and generally enhance the quality of your life. What makes them beneficial is that they work in harmony with the body. Each oil has the ability to evoke different memories that can affect the physical, emotional, and psychological levels of a person. Best of all, using essential oils boosts the immune system by combating the stress that ultimately weakens the body's resistance and makes you susceptible to illness.

Scents can trigger memories due to their quick access to the limbic system in the brain. It is here that scents will trigger an emotional response, such as hunger or sexual appetite. They can help you recall long- and short-term memories. If a particular scent stirs up past hurts, painful emotions and memories, and causes you suffering, then you might want to avoid this specific scent. But I believe that it is good to be able to release this kind of hurt and pain rather than avoid it. Think about the scents that can bring about recollection of your past experiences; smells spur memories.

Extraction Methods

Essential oils can be found in all the various parts of a plant, their seeds, roots, bark, leaves, wood, balsam, resin, and flowers. The art of their extraction has developed slowly over time, and many new techniques are becoming available. It takes a large quantity of plant material to make a small amount of essential oil; for instance, it can take 1 ton of rose petals to produce 10½ ounces of rose oil.

Maceration is the oldest method of producing an "infused oil." This process, which softens the plant materials by steeping, produces a liquid that has absorbed some of the plant's therapeutic benefits.

Distillation is a process in which plant material fills huge vats and is steamed at high pressure. The heat and steam cause the cell structure of the plant material to burst and break down, freeing the essential oils. The vapor is then cooled, condensed, and collected. This is the most popular method by which essential oils are obtained from plants.

Expression, in which the peel of a fruit is squeezed, is a process reserved for obtaining citrus oils.

How to Purchase and Store

Essential oils are extremely precious and should be treated with respect. They also vary in cost depending on the plant; I purposely eliminated jasmine and rose from the recipe bath blends because they can be much more costly. While the lavender plant produces more oil, rose or jasmine produces a very small amount, and that affects the price.

When you have chosen which bath you would like to experience, purchase the particular essential oils listed for it. Make sure the oils come in either brown or cobalt blue glass bottles; the coloring protects them from decomposition caused by ultraviolet light. Purchase the smallest size bottles to keep your expenses down until you discover your favorite bath blend combinations.

The experienced aromatherapist can tell just by smelling the oil if it is of a higher quality or if it has been diluted with a carrier oil — such as jojoba, grapeseed, or apricot — that is used to dilute a pure essential oil so it can be used in a massage or perfume blend. Quality depends also on the method of processing and extraction: how and where the plant was grown, and if the right amount of pressure and steam was used during its distillation. Just keep in mind that essential oils do vary tremendously, but you will still reap the benefits.

You might find oils or products that are labeled ESSENCE. These are chemically synthesized. You *do not* want these; although they might smell nice, they do not have the medicinal properties necessary for the baths.You should purchase only products marked PURE ESSENTIAL OILS and check the origin of the brand. Inhale some essential oils sold in health-food stores and pharmacies and buy those that immediately appeal to you. Let your nose guide you.

Keep the essential oil bottles away from heat, stored in a cool, dark place. This will prolong their shelf life. The optimum shelf life of an essential oil is about one year. After this time some of the oils start losing their potency, but the time period varies depending on the oil.

Making Personal Scents

When you have experienced a bath blend that I've recommended, you might feel a personal, intuitive connection with it and may want to expand on the use of it throughout the day. You can make a perfume oil by using my bath dosage, then adding it to a carrier oil such as grapeseed or jojoba oil (available in health-food stores). To every 100 drops of carrier oil, add my recommended essential oil dosage. If you like the blend enough to use it daily as a perfume, dilute it with 50 drops of vodka. Vodka has no scent and acts like an alcohol perfume dilutant; it will evaporate on your skin, leaving only the essential oil fragrance. Your own natural body scent will be enhanced and not masked, and the oil will be absorbed through your skin via the bloodstream and through olfaction.

Blending Oils

When I embark on the adventure of making even the simplest blend, I eagerly anticipate the final product. Start with a cleared-off space such as a kitchen counter or table. Cover the surface where you are placing the open bottles of essential oil; any spillage can damage the surface of your table. I use a marble lazy Susan to protect my tabletop.

Most essential oils have little plastic covers that allow only a drop at a time to come out, but if this is not the case, you can purchase disposable plastic eyedroppers or reusable glass ones very inexpensively for this use. Keep your different oil droppers separate; if you use a dropper for one oil and then use it for another, it can alter the blend. Instead, clean reusable droppers with rubbing alcohol and let them dry thoroughly. You also can soak them in vodka.

Most health-food stores carry "treatment bottles" for Bach flower remedies that are empty, amber-colored glass and have their own eyedroppers. They come in a box of four for only $1.50. I find these most appropriate and affordable, and excellent for storage. A blend will keep for about three to six months if it is stored in an amber-colored bottle in a cool place away from sunlight. Storing for a longer period can cause deterioration of the rubber bulb on the dropper.

Once you've put the recommended dosages in the bottle and closed the cap tightly, swish the bottle around to blend the oils very gently, rather than in a vigorous manner. Remember: They are precious substances and energies that should be appreciated. When I am creating blends, I feel like a perfumer and chemist, making magic potions derived from an ancient time. Treat your blend as if it were liquid gold.

Remember to practice blending as often as you can and you will start to incorporate aromatherapy into your life on a daily basis. Be very patient with yourself, as you will then start to become familiar with the subtle effects of each essential oil.

Oils to Avoid during Pregnancy or If You Have Asthma

Although many essential oils are perfectly safe for use during pregnancy, some should be avoided. Do not use the following oils if you are pregnant or even might be. Also, do not use the bath blends if you are pregnant unless recommended by a qualified health care practitioner. These oils can irritate the respiratory tract, so avoid them if you have asthma.

Essential Oil	Botanical Name	Essential Oil	Botanical Name
Aniseed	*Pimpinella anisum*	Lavender*	*Lavandula officinalis*
Anjelica	*Angelica archangelica*	Marjoram*	*Origanum majorana*
		Myrrh	*Commiphora myrrha*
Basil	*Ocimum basilicum*		
Bergamot	*Citrus aurantium bergamia*	Neroli*	*Citrus aurantium*
		Nutmeg	*Myristica fragrans*
Cedarwood	*Cedrus atlantica*	Patchouli	*Pogostemon patchouli*
Citronella	*Cymbopogon nardus*		
		Peppermint	*Mentha x piperita*
Clary sage	*Salvia sclarea*	Rosemary	*Rosmarinus officinalis*
Clove	*Eugenia caryophyllata*		
		Sandalwood	*Santalum album*
Cumin	*Cuminum cyminum*	Thyme	*Thymus vulgaris*
Fennel	*Foeniculum vulgare*	Ylang ylang	*Cananga odorata*

* See box, below.

Safe Oils for Asthmatics

The essential oils useful for reducing the anxiety of asthma attacks and improving the function of lungs are cypress, lavender, marjoram, frankincense, melissa, neroli, Roman chamomile, and rose. A blend of these oils can be massaged into the chest and upper back. Putting 1 drop of essential oil on a cotton ball and inhaling also helps. If you suffer from asthma, consult with an experienced aromatherapist before trying to create your own blends.

Special Selected Oils and Their Properties

These essential oils are fairly inexpensive, widely available, and very versatile in bath blends. You should be familiar with the effect that each oil produces.

Cautions on the Use of Essential Oils

The oils I have recommended in this book have been carefully selected for their gentle healing properties. Adhere to my dosage instructions! Discontinue use if any irritation arises. When you are working with different essential oils, try not to expose yourself to too many of them at once for a prolonged period. I have found myself "scent-sory" overloaded from working with too many fragrances. Your body will tell you if you are overdoing it; you might get a headache or feel a little nauseous.

Pure essential oil can irritate or burn the skin, so use caution in handling. If you do experience irritation, rub pure carrier oil — such as jojoba, apricot, safflower, canola, grapeseed, or olive — onto the skin to dilute the oil. Be very careful not to rub your eyes after handling oil. Note, also, that any spillage on clothing will stain like perfume or other oil-based product. And always keep essential oils out of the reach of children.

Bergamot

Bergamot essential oil is used to treat depression, anxiety, and stress-related conditions. It is very uplifting and sweetly fragrant. The highest quality of this essential oil comes from Reggio di Calabria, located in southern Italy, although the oil itself is named after the Italian city of Bergamo in Lombardy. Here it was used for many years to treat fever, malaria, worms, and respiratory and urinary tract infections.

The bergamot tree, *Citrus aurantium bergamia,* belongs to the cultivated hybrid of bitter orange and lemon. It grows to about 16 feet high, yet appears to be more fragile than an orange or a lemon tree. The trees have green leaves with small, white, star-shaped flowers that have a sweet smell.

The essential oil is usually made from the incredibly bitter green fruit, which is so sour that it is inedible. The skin of this fruit has small oil glands that hold the highly valued ingredient.

The application of bergamot is most enjoyable to me in the summer, when I make an after-shower splash that leaves me sweet and clean smelling. To make your own, add 4 to 6 drops of essential oil to 1 quart of room temperature distilled water; shake well. Splash on your damp body and allow your skin to air dry. You will feel balanced and uplifted.

Freshen the Carpet with Essential Oil?

Before vacuuming the carpet, place about 10 drops of your favorite essential oil on a small scrap of cloth and toss it into the bag. Especially energizing fragrances like peppermint and eucalyptus will not only help you get the job done sooner, but will also leave the carpet smelling fresh. I also take a small square of fabric and put about 8 to 10 drops of an essential oil like lavender or bergamot or lemon and toss it into the dryer, so the clothes and linens smell naturally fresh, clean, and sweetly scented.

Clary Sage

Clary sage is related to the mint family. It is cultivated today in Russia, France, Spain, and Italy. This plant, *Salvia sclarea,* grows up to 4 feet high and has large green, hairy leaves with tiny blue flowers. Centuries ago the clary sage plant was used to increase the intoxicating effects of inferior wine and beer. The essential oil is euphoric and intoxicating and should not be used while drinking alcohol; it can induce a narcotic effect and exaggerate drunkenness! It has a warm, sweet fragrance that is helpful for treating nervousness, stress, fear, paranoia, anxiety, and depression.

Clary sage oil also induces creativity and inspiration when you feel a "mental block"; it will also help maintain mental clarity. When used in a diffuser, clary sage essential oil aids in easing tightness in the bronchial tubes resulting from colds and bronchitis. This oil is soothing yet uplifting, and makes a good relaxing aphrodisiac that will ease impotence and frigidity. It is very beneficial for PMS symptoms if used in a bath or massage.

Lavender

The scent of lavender is familiar to everyone. *Lavandula officinalis* originally grew in the high mountains of Persia and southern France. An evergreen shrub, it reaches up to 3 feet in height and has beautiful violet flowers. France produces a thousand tons of lavender oil each year.

The healing power of lavender is extremely diverse. It was used in Persia, Greece, and Rome to disinfect hospital and sickrooms. During the Great Plague, lavender was part of a mixture called Four Thieves Vinegar, used successfully by grave robbers to avoid contracting the deadly disease. The botanical name *Lavandula* comes from the Latin word *lavare,* meaning "to wash." It is a pure clean fragrance that seems to wash away impurities in the body and mind.

I use this essential oil when treating psychological problems such as nervousness, insomnia, stress, depression, melancholy, fear, and irritability. It stimulates and regenerates the nervous system and brings a feeling of calm. Many people now use lavender oil and tea to help relieve headache; you can massage a couple of drops of the oil into the temples, or inhale the fragrance directly from the bottle. If you find the smell of a bottle of lavender oil too strong, put 3 drops on a cotton ball and inhale the scent. It is a wonderful relaxer. Lavender oil also stimulates white blood cell formation and therefore strengthens the body's immune system.

In France some people inhale small amounts of lavender oil when they get a cold, influenza, or bronchitis. But lavender is also helpful for treating high blood pressure and strengthening the heart. In ancient Rome, housewives put lavender between freshly washed linens in the drawers and chests. Moths hate the scent!

Marjoram

The ancient Greeks used marjoram in their medicines, cosmetics, and fragrances. The word "marjoram" is derived from the Greek word *morosganos,* meaning "joy of the mountains." Marjoram was given to a newly married couple as a token of good luck, and was even planted in graveyards to assist in bringing peace to the departed spirit. It is very helpful for muscular pain, bruises, and stiff joints.

Origanum majorana is native to the Mediterranean region, Egypt, and North Africa. Its fragrance is warm and spicy and very calming. It is helpful during anxiety attacks, tension, stress, grief, depression, and insomnia. Marjoram can lower high blood pressure and ease migraine headaches. Because the oil stimulates menstruation, it should not be used during pregnancy.

Disinfectant Room Spray

Try this blend to make a healthy, fragrant room spray that also has disinfectant properties.

15 drops lavender

8 drops lemon

2 drops eucalyptus

2 ounces distilled water

Add the essential oils to the water in a spritzer bottle (available at drugstores). Shake well before each spray: the oil blend floats right to the top of the water.

Myrrh

This oil is spicy, dark, and reddish brown in color. The tree, *Commiphora myrrha,* can grow up to 33 feet high, with knotted branches, aromatic leaves, and white flowers. It grows in northeast Africa, southwest Asia, and Ethiopia. This substance has been used in magic and religion for about 4,000 years. In Egypt, for example, myrrh was used to make incense and to pack the body cavities during the embalming process.

Myrrh is mentioned in the Bible, along with gold and frankincense, as one of the gifts the wise men brought to the baby Jesus. The Greeks used it as an antiseptic and skin healing agent. According to Greek mythology, Myrrha refused to worship Aphrodite, the goddess of love. The goddess was so angry that she threatened to have Myrrha killed. The other gods felt sorry for Myrrha, so they changed her into a "weeping" tree. The gum resin from this tree falls in tear-shaped drops.

I breathe in myrrh, sandalwood, or frankincense prior to meditation. It expands my awareness and allows me to go deeper inside myself. Myrrh is a known sedative. It also increases confidence, and helps you to move through obstacles.

Neroli (Orange Blossom)

This oil has a beautiful smell with the delicate freshness of a warm, sweet, floral fragrance. It was named after a princess of Nerola, in Italy, who wore it as her signature perfume. Neroli has many uses, including as an aphrodisiac and antidepressant, for anxiety and nervous tension relief, as a euphoric, and as a treatment for several stress-related disorders.

Neroli essential oil is obtained from the fragrant white blossoms of the Seville orange tree, *Citrus aurantium*. One ton of freshly picked flowers is required to produce 16 ounces of oil, making it one of the most precious oils. The flowers were used in bridal bouquets to calm anxiety before the honeymoon night and to inspire abundance and fertility.

I use neroli oil for self-purification. Inhale the scent while visualizing it burning away negative thought patterns and bad habits; it will help you feel more joyful. Just sniff the scent to lift your spirits and settle your emotions. Neroli oil can even create a feeling of euphoria. In addition, it calms the mind of worries over sexual performance.

Peppermint

Peppermint oil is excellent for mental fatigue and stress. Inhaling its scent will also ease migraines and encourage concentration. This herb is a native of Europe, but the main producer of peppermint is now the United States. *Mentha* x *piperita* grows about 3 feet high and has purple spiked flowers and serrated leaves that are slightly hairy.

The Romans would crown themselves with peppermint at feasts, aware of its detoxifying effects; it was even used in wine to prevent hangovers! It has been used in Eastern and Western medicine for relieving nausea, indigestion, sore throat, diarrhea, headache, and toothache. This tasty plant even helps relieve morning sickness and dysmenorrhea.

Peppermint tea is quite popular; peppermint is also an ingredient in cold and cough remedies. You've tasted it in chewing gum, mouthwash, alcoholic beverages, and soft drinks, and smelled it in tobacco, perfumes, and cosmetics. It is very useful for inhalation in asthma. Because peppermint is stimulating, it should not be used at night or you'll wind up staying up later than you might like!

Patchouli

The word patchouli is from the Hindustani and has a very long history of being used medicinally in China, Malaysia, India, and Japan. In Victorian times, the dried leaves of *Pogostemon patchouli* were placed within the folds of Indian cashmere shawls to protect them from moths. It was also used in sachets to perfume linen and keep away "bed bugs." The scent of patchouli is used to arouse sexual desire and has been celebrated as an aphrodisiac for more than a century. This versatile plant oil is also reputed to manifest money. Put a few drops of the dark oil on a cotton ball, inhale, and visualize!

When I wear patchouli oil, it is immediately recognizable to others. It gets mixed reactions: Most people love it, but some are repulsed by it. After a few minutes, I can't even smell it on myself, but others do — so use it sparingly! If you need a quick start in the morning, sniff the oil for a second or two.

The properties of patchouli are antidepressant, antiseptic, aphrodisiac, astringent, deodorant, sedative (in low doses), and stimulant (in high doses). It increases the libido by its bracing action on the central nervous system. It is said to regenerate tissue by helping the regrowth of skin cells and forming scar tissue. It heals rough, cracked skin, sores, wounds, and acne. Even better, patchouli oil is grounding and balancing.

Rosemary

The botanical name, *Rosmarinus officinalis,* comes from the Latin *rosmarinus,* or "sea dew," for the plant's fondness of water. Though originally from Asia, much rosemary essential oil now is obtained from France and Tunisia. Traces of rosemary have even been found in

Egyptian tombs. The Greeks and Romans used it as incense to drive away evil spirits. The queen of Hungary, Dona Isabella, used it as a face wash to restore her youthful looks. Its antiseptic properties were used in French hospitals, where it was burned during epidemics.

Rosemary is known as a restorative, stimulating circulation, brain function, and sexual desire. I use it to clear my mind and help my memory. It enlivens the brain cells because it is invigorating and strengthening — perfect for when you are feeling exhausted. It relieves tired muscles, rheumatic pain, poor circulation, asthma, and stress-related disorders. In some cultures, rosemary is also used in bridal wreaths to promote lasting love.

When you need to memorize something, put a few drops of rosemary essential oil on a cotton ball next to you and sniff it as you study. Then when you are actually taking the test, smell the essential oil again and the information will come to you.

For matters of the heart, inhale the scent of rosemary oil and strongly visualize it bringing love into your life; smell it throughout the day. You can also smell rosemary oil and visualize a long, healthy life.

Sandalwood

Sandalwood is derived from the Sanskrit word *chandara*. With sandalwood, you will experience a warmth and balance that will fill your heart with joy. It has a warm and spicy fragrance that helps to release you from tension, confusion, and anxiety, bringing calmness to your soul.

This exotic essential oil captures the mystery of Asia, where it is part of ayurveda, the Indian system of healing. It was used in embalming and for funeral rituals for princes to help free the soul in death. Even today, the wood is burned on a sacred fire within a marriage tent so its fumes surround a Hindu couple for love and good fortune.

In Burma, women sprinkle people walking by with a mixture of rose water and sandalwood oil on the last day of the year to wash away their sins for the new year. Sandalwood is useful for aiding meditation and for religious ceremonies, and is still popular in India and China. The Egyptians used it in embalming and as a remedy for gonorrhea because it had a cleansing action on the sexual organs.

Sandalwood originated in India, in the state of Karnataka. The *Santalum album* tree grows 30 feet high, and the wood is yellowish. The essential oil is derived from the wood of the tree by steam distillation. This versatile oil is used as an antiseptic, cramp reliever, aphrodisiac, and to quiet irritated emotions. It is also very good for stress, depression, tension, insomnia, impotence, frigidity, and aggression. Remember to use at your own discretion — the properties of this aphrodisiac are well known!

Sandalwood is one of my favorite essential oils. Be aware that the sandalwood tree is endangered; cherish its oil, and use it responsibly.

A Natural Attractant

Sandalwood has long been considered an aphrodisiac. Scientists have researched old applications of sandalwood and discovered a connection with the erotic quality of the oil. Men's underarm perspiration releases androsterone, a hormone that is similar in its chemical structure and components to the male hormone testosterone. Androsterone smells similar to sandalwood, which sends out barely perceivable erotic signals to the opposite sex.

Thyme

The fragrance of thyme is hot, herbal, and intense. The translation of the Greek word for thyme is "courage"; it supplies energy in times of psychological and physical weakness. This popular herb helps to restore and build strength during illness. It increases intelligence and memory and helps in concentration. Thyme is also used to relieve blockages caused by past traumas.

As an antibacterial, thyme works to break down the bacteria's enzymes. Thyme destroys *Staphylococcus* even after the essential oil has been diluted more than 1,000 times! By increasing the formation of white blood cells, thyme is very effective in combating viruses; inhalation of the essential oil helps protect against infections and diseases. It is a disinfectant, and also an antispasmodic for colds, flu, bronchitis, and sinusitis. This oil is used in mouthwashes, gargles, toothpaste, and lozenges.

The Egyptians used thyme effectively in embalming. It was also used to ward off infection, paralysis, multiple sclerosis, and leprosy. Thyme should not be used if you have high blood pressure, however, but it is said to be helpful in childbirth to speed up delivery and to expel the afterbirth. It has a cleansing action that helps after miscarriage. This oil, from the *Thymus vulgaris* plant, strengthens you mentally, emotionally, and physically.

Ylang Ylang

Cananga odorata, the ylang ylang tree, originated in the Philippines and is now also cultivated in Java, Sumatra, Madagascar, Zanzibar, and Haiti. This tree grows up to 66 feet high. The blooms are unusually large, with yellowish white petals and a strong, sweet scent. The flower blossoms need to be harvested in the early-morning hours in order to produce the highest quality oil. This is one of my favorite oils and I use it with regularity.

This essential oil stimulates the part of the brain that releases endorphins. It creates a euphoric and erotic mood. Ylang ylang is a very intense oil that I find myself magnetically drawn to when I need a powerful jolt to change my mood. I get giddy with repeated applications! Its scent takes me to faraway lands that only my imagination has traveled to. If it is too sweet for you, tone it down with orange or lemon essential oil.

Ylang ylang has the extraordinary ability to relax your facial muscles. It calms anger and other negative emotional states, transforming the energy into a more positive one. But I like it so much because it activates my enthusiasm. Wear it or inhale it prior to all nerve-racking situations such as job interviews or any dreaded event. As you breathe it in, visualize the essential oil energy doing its work and you will get through the event just fine. On special occasions, when I'm serving my visitors champagne, I've added 3 drops of ylang ylang to the bottle before pouring. My guests enjoy the special effects of the subtle, subliminal flavor that it induces: joy!

Inhaling ylang ylang and using the appropriate visualization make for a powerful aphrodisiac. In Indonesia, the flowers are spread on the bed of newlyweds. In the Victorian age, ylang ylang was used to prevent fever, fight infections, and as a hair conditioner. It relieves depression, frigidity, impotence, insomnia, nervousness, and stress.

Bath Preparation

To make your bath the most beneficial and enjoyable experience possible, prepare in advance so that you don't have to rush around. Here are a few basic guidelines:

1. Wait a couple of hours after eating to take your bath. This will allow you time to digest, and will facilitate your mind and body in achieving the full effect.
2. Rewrite each of the mental exercises on index cards in bold print or photocopy them for quick reference while in the bath. Cover the cards with clear tape or insert them into a plastic photo pocket to waterproof so that they can be wiped dry for later use.
3. Have a nice fluffy towel ready for you after your bath.
4. Place a good no-slip rug by the tub to step onto upon exiting.
5. Drink a glass of *room temperature* spring water before entering the bath and immediately after exiting.

Beauty and the Bath: Creating a "Sacred Space"

Ideally your bathroom should be both a refuge from the turmoil and tensions of the outside world and a place of warmth and welcome. It should be a supportive environment in which you can accomplish your meditative aromatherapy baths in privacy and peace. With little effort you can create a much more relaxing atmosphere. First, you need to make it visually relaxing. Clear out the clutter! Keep it clean and fresh smelling. Throw damp towels that are hanging on the shower rod or on doorknobs into the dryer and out of sight. Your bathroom can become your personal space.

In creating your "sacred space," select and display objects of art and nature, or even candles, that will add to the environment in an inviting way. Hang up inspiring art in unusual frames that personalize your space, no matter how small your bathroom or budget. For years I've collected interesting bottles, crystal bowls, silver trays for scented soaps, bath oils, salts, potpourri, and candles. I have unusual seashells from my travels. On my bathroom walls I have framed watercolors of cavorting dolphins with the ocean in the background that I bought in St. Lucia on my honeymoon.

Another favorite is an antique colored champagne glass in which I keep fresh lavender and tiny rosebuds, and I freshen them with a few drops of lavender essential oil. Select pictures and other objects that connect with you. You can find interesting and exotic bottles at thrift shops and antique stores. You can purchase unscented bath salts and scent them with your favorite essential oil. The more attention paid to this room, the more inviting it will become for you.

The bath is a special sanctuary from the troubles of our existence. It is a place to relax, to meditate, to let go of disturbing thoughts. Transform your experience and increase your degree of pleasure by adding the essential oils I recommend. Allow the aromas to envelop your body, mind, and spirit.

Bring Nature Indoors

Houseplants and flowers enhance the beauty and tranquillity of your home, including your bathroom. I always keep a small bunch of fresh flowers by the bathroom sink. Because I have a special emotional connection to gardenias, which were also my mother's favorite flowers, I like to keep a plant nearby. I also float them in crystal bowls of water in the bathroom.

Select plants for their ability to thrive indoors, especially plants that enjoy the humidity of the bathroom. Avoid toxic plants if you have children and pets. Green and silver foliage is very relaxing, while the reds and purples are more stimulating. It is also important to know the amount of natural light and temperature they require for their survival, so check with a nursery salesperson before choosing your plants. The Chinese believe that the cactus brings luck to the home, but you wouldn't want to back into one of these while naked!

Above all, make sure you will remain undisturbed for the duration of the bathing process. It is important that all daily activities be put on hold so you can devote your full attention to each mental exercise. This is not only quality time, it is also sacred time, time for you.

Entering and Emerging from the Bath

Add the selected oils *after* you have run a full warm bath, then stir to make sure the oil is evenly dispersed. Plan to remain in the tub for at least 20 minutes.

Light a candle of the correct color for your particular mood choice. Do not step into the tub until the bath is fully drawn. Once the bath is prepared, remind yourself that it is your time to reaffirm faith in yourself and the connection to your spiritual and emotional center. Use caution entering and exiting the tub; sit on the edge of the tub and slide in. Slide down and, on your back, submerge the face, leaving the nose and mouth out of the water. You should stay in this position for as long as it takes to complete the accompanying exercise.

Allow your body to relax in the scented water. Be sure to immerse your scalp to achieve the full benefits of the aromatherapeutic experience. Breathe in the aromas through your nose, hold it, then breathe out through your mouth. Take nice, long, deep breaths. Do this three times. Now you are ready to begin your visualization. Follow the guided imagery, meditation, or affirmation given with that particular bath. And enjoy the exquisite transformation!

When ready, emerge from the tub. Don't rush. Cover yourself in a soft towel; blot, don't rub, your skin. Alternatively, you could allow your skin to air dry.

The reaction to each bath is highly individualized, but the combination of using the power of your mind with the power of essential oils can produce incredible results. You might emerge with more clarity and insight, deep relaxation, profound peace, and feeling lighter. Always block out time for you to be alone and introspective after a healing bath.

Bath Tips

Essential oil baths have a cleansing action that elicits a physical, emotional, mental, and spiritual response. It might take a little time before you see significant results, but the more you practice, the more you allow a deeper connection with your inner persona to develop.

There isn't a special time of day that is best for a bath; the best time is when you know you won't be interrupted or get distracted because you have to rush off somewhere. The fewer distractions, the better your concentration will be. It is preferred that the bathroom be warm because your body temperature decreases while meditating. Turn up the heat or shut the windows, if you wish; you will distract yourself if you have to run hot water.

Try to space the baths at least two days apart if you are working with different moods. You can do the same bath every day for 7 to 10 days. Light a candle or dim the lights for ambience, but *do not fall asleep!*

What If I Don't Like Baths?

If you are not a bath person and prefer showers, you can still enjoy the healing effects of an aromatherapy blend. Make up the bath blend in advance by using the designated amounts of the essential oils, and put them in a plastic spray bottle filled with 4 ounces of distilled water or spring water. After showering, spray yourself with the blend, avoiding the genital area. Close your eyes and allow your skin to air dry. While lying in bed in a quiet room, practice the deep breathing that is suggested for the bath, then follow with the accompanying meditation and visualization.

Enhancing Your Life with Aromatherapy

It really is so simple to bring aromatherapy into your life, and once you start to bathe in the beauty of nature and open the doors to healing, you will bring more quality to your existence. The day I stepped into the world of aromatherapy, my life was completely transformed. I hope that my suggestions and experiences will encourage, inspire, and teach you a new way of healing.

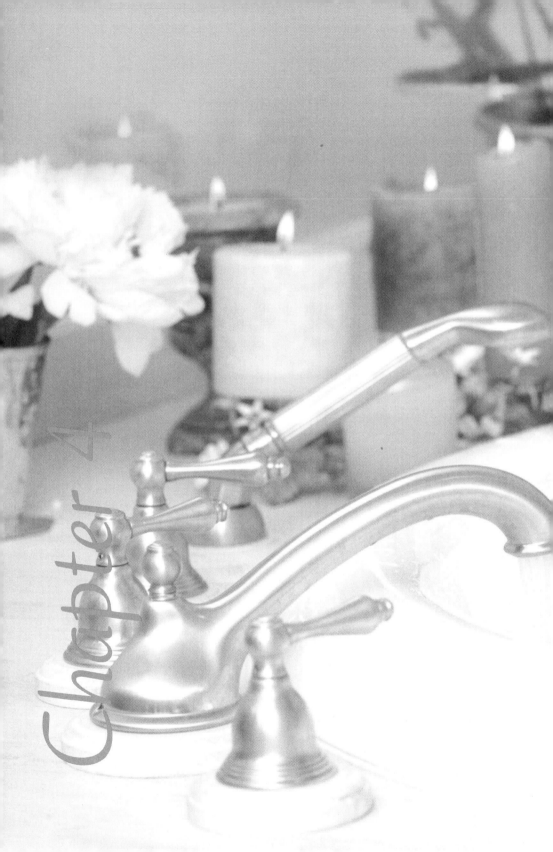

Chapter 4

Using Color Therapy

Color synchronizes the different parts of your brain. The reticular activating system (RAS) is the section of the brain that receives sensory input and tells us either to calm down or to prepare to fight or run. It is essential for our survival, but if this system is overactive, it can block feelings of peace and tranquillity. If you think of a relaxing experience, the RAS responds by calming you down.

Color works in the same way. Colors like blue, green, and violet subconsciously relax you, thereby affecting your state of mind. Our internal vibrations — our life-force energy, or what is known in Asian philosophy as *prana* or *chi* — flow freely through us and make us feel whole and connected. When our internal vibrations are in harmony with the world and with the people in our lives, we are healthier and have a higher energy level. Vibrational healing systems from color therapy introduce harmonious energies into the system so any imbalance can be corrected.

Using Color to Heal

The color spectrum can be divided into eight main hues: red, orange, yellow, green, turquoise, blue, violet, and magenta. When we work with colors, our bodies become sensitive to them. This then enables us to feel the vibrational frequency of each color.

Even the color of clothes we wear has an effect on us, not just emotionally but also physically. When I wear yellow it is usually because I need a mood lift that day. I feel brighter, cheerier, as if the color has seeped into my pores. When I choose to wear aqua, I feel more serene, like the sea goddess Yemaya, more connected to the ocean and nature. Have you ever noticed when shopping for a new blouse or shirt that even if you like the style, a particular color can cause a slight shiver or distasteful reaction? Or perhaps you might be drawn to the shade but are disappointed by the style. Every morning, when selecting what to wear for the day, I pay attention to what the color of each garment does for me.

Color is used in meditation and visualization for the purpose of healing. Each color vibration has its own wavelength and frequency for healing action on a cellular level. Each gland and body organ has a vibrational frequency sympathetic to one of the colors; your cells vibrate at the same frequency as one of the colors. As pioneering German educator and philosopher Rudolf Steiner pointed out, cells are light sensitive, so when light vibrations reach the cells either through the eyes or the skin, chemical changes occur that affect the growth and behavior of those cells. In this way, the DNA within the cells resonates to different light frequencies, or colors. Through Steiner's work, it became accepted that color has a profound effect on both the mind and the body.

In a famous study, it was discovered that an infant's bedroom painted yellow — an uplifting color that should not be used where a state of relaxation is desired — caused such anxiety that there was an increase in the amount of crying. In color therapy, vibrational healing systems of color induce harmonious vibrations into the body so that balance and the flow of energy can be restored. The vibrations of color disperse blocked energy that is within our emotional, mental, and spiritual bodies.

Specific Color Details

Each color has its own frequency and wavelength. The longest wavelength and shortest frequency is red, and as you go down the color spectrum, magenta has the shortest wavelength and highest frequency. When you work with color, your body becomes sensitive to it, and more open to meditation and healing. Color affects you physically, psychologically, and emotionally. In order for you to appreciate the power of color, it is important to know each color's attributes.

Red increases vitality and energy. This color is traditionally the seat of life-force energy; it is invigorating, vital, activating.

Orange is cheerful, working as an antidepressant and creating a happy environment. Use orange when you need to facilitate the process of letting go. Relaxation of mind and body and loosening areas of stress can be attained with orange.

Yellow has a detaching quality, creating a lack of involvement. It is uplifting, but a large amount of the hue induces nervousness and tension, and can be disorienting or perplexing. This color has been known to distort perspective.

Green can cause hyperactivity without scattering your energy. Green promotes sound judgment, stability, and physical equilibrium.

Turquoise is soothing, inviting interest and easing tension. This color helps release anxiety while providing support. Turquoise is refreshing and stimulating; it is best used in the bedroom and office.

Blue is a relaxing color. It invites communication, meditation, and balance by calming the body and mind. Because blue creates softness, it is best used in stress-related areas such as the office.

Violet promotes self-confidence and a love and concern for others. Use violet in meditation and prayer, when you need to concentrate. It is the center of self-respect and pride and expresses individuality. Inner balance, silence, and relaxation are all aided by violet. A mind-balancing color, it helps you unburden and protect yourself. But violet is also an aphrodisiac, and is widely used in areas of festivity.

Magenta helps raise energy levels. This color is impervious and forceful, and is used to stimulate. Magenta brings self-respect, dignity, and composure by aiding concentration. It is also the color of spiritual love.

Simple Ways to Incorporate Color into Your Healing

Even today, the ancient Indian system of solar-ray healing still recommends therapeutic color baths. To make your own therapeutic color bath, purchase a colored lightbulb in the shade you need to evoke a mood. Avoid fluorescent lights; they emit pulsing flickers that can make you ill. Insert the colored bulb into your bathroom fixture or portable lamp and light it for use during your bath. Of course, if you are using a portable lamp, be sure it is a safe distance from water.

Colors for Healing

The following healing color list should be used in visualization exercises to help restore your well-being.

Color	Used to Treat
Red	anemia, cold, leukemia, numbness
Orange	agoraphobia, alcoholism, arthritis, common cold, constipation, depression, fatigue, gallstones, gout, kidney disease, liver disease, rheumatism, muscular stiffness, ulcers
Yellow	arthritis, hepatitis, jaundice, rheumatism
Green	angina, chest pain, gastric ulcer, heart disease, peptic ulcer, trauma, tumors, warts
Turquoise	abscess, acne, asthma, boils, cold sore, dermatitis, eczema, fatigue, fever, hay fever, pneumonia, stings, stress, swelling, tension
Blue	anxiety, acne, asthma, backache, blisters, bruises, burns, cough, cramp, dermatitis,earache, emphysema, flatulence, gallstones, German measles, glandular fever, hay fever, hernia, herpes, hiccups, influenza, itching, laryngitis, lumbago, mumps, PMS, sneezing, sores, sprains, stammering, stiffness, stings, stress, sunburn, tonsillitis, toothache, wheezing
Violet	conjunctivitis, earache, menopause, mental illness, myopia, neuralgia, paranoia, warts
Magenta	fainting, headache, migraine, morning sickness, nausea, shock, stroke, vomiting

I like to use natural food coloring in my bathwater. Several drops added to the bath won't affect your skin and will tint the water to a gentle hue. A handful of fresh flowers provides you with a color energy bath. Leave the blossoms to float around the surface of the water so they can visually stimulate you, rather than tying them up in a bag.

Candles are many people's favorite bath accessory. They are soothing and beautiful, and help bring a sense of peace to the room. Choose candles in colors that promote the desired mood.

Chapter 5

the
Stress
Relief
Bath

The more you know about stress, the better equipped you will be to minimize stress-related problems. Stress can not only ruin your day, but doctors are discovering that it can also ruin your health. When we are faced with a stressful situation, impulses are sent to the brain via the nervous system that activate the pituitary gland to secrete hormones into the bloodstream. These hormones activate the adrenal glands to secrete adrenaline and noradrenaline. This increases your blood sugar. Research has proved that when your tissues are soaked in stress hormones, your blood pressure, blood sugar, and heart rate skyrocket, while your capability for digestion and absorption shuts down.

Chronic stress increases your risk of everything from glaucoma to heart disease, and makes you 50 percent more likely to catch the latest virus going around. Studies have shown that at least 80 percent of doctor's visits are for health problems that have been triggered by stress!

What Is Stress?

Stress can be caused by a multitude of life imbalances, such as job dissatisfaction, a strained marital relationship, and illness in the family. But even a smaller problem — for instance, a public presentation, a flat tire, or a missed appointment — can cause stress. Studies have shown that even those people with a longer commute to work (45 minutes or more) experience more stress than those with a shorter daily trip!

The first stage is the alarm reaction. Your brain signals your nervous system and your endocrine system to get various parts of the body ready to cope with the emergency. These are the responses of your body to the first stage of stress:

~ The motor nerves prepare the muscles in your arms and legs for motion ("fight or flight").
~ Your blood pressure, heart rate, and blood sugar levels go up.

~ Adrenaline is released into the bloodstream as a stimulant.
~ The skin receives decreased blood flow, which can lead to cold hands and feet, high blood pressure, and migraine headaches.

Your body can't maintain the alarm level of arousal forever, so after severe or repeated stress, you come to the stage of exhaustion. The long-term effects of stress on the heart range from rapid beating, pounding, and irregular beats to angina and coronary artery disease.

STRESS RELIEF BLEND

Soak away anxiety and stress with this bath. The most relaxing baths are warm, not hot! Hot water shocks the system, causing muscles to contract. Warm water calms you by increasing circulation and relaxing the muscles. Do not use the bath if you are asthmatic or pregnant but perform the accompanying visualization.

3 drops bergamot essential oil

2 drops clary sage essential oil

2 drops sandalwood essential oil

2 drops neroli essential oil

2 drops lavender essential oil

Stress Relief

Close your eyes and simply take a deep breath, being aware of the exquisite natural extracts you are breathing in. Breathe in calmness and exhale tension. Breathe with your belly, imagining that your lungs are sitting right behind your belly button. In order to fill them with air, relax your abdomen and let it expand with each breath. Slowly inhale for a count of 8, filling your belly, and slowly exhale to the count of 8.

Do a few repetitions of this and then concentrate on each area of your body, starting with the top of the head, and release the tension from your muscles one by one, all the way down to your toes and back up again. Continue to breathe in relaxation and exhale all the tension.

Now that your body feels soft and relaxed, allow your awareness to come inside yourself. Visualize yourself walking on a path among trees . . . walking in a place in nature. In front of you is a gate. Open the gate and step into a beautiful garden.

You see and smell the most beautiful flowers you have ever seen. You see lush palm trees and fruit trees and tropical flowers perfumed with sweet fragrances. Touch them . . . smell them . . . inhale the aromas. Each time you inhale, you feel more calm and relaxed. Listen to the singing birds. Feel the calm, gentle breeze; it is a celebration of nature in its magnificent form.

A wonderful feeling of peace and joy drifts through your mind and flows through your body. Visualize a magnificent cool waterfall. As you step into it, feel the cool, clean, refreshing water cascade upon you, cleansing you from the top of your head down to your toes, washing away every bit of stress and anxiety. Allow your being to be restored on all levels.

Now project your thoughts forward. In a vision, see yourself in what might be a stressful situation, but as you see this vision, allow the exquisite feeling of relaxation to continue to soothe your thoughts. Allow the relaxed state you are feeling now to weave a tapestry of a totally stress-free consciousness into your vision. Your mind and body are being conditioned to respond calmly, peacefully to stress.

Open your eyes slowly, taking with you this calm and relaxing feeling, remembering you can always return to this peaceful garden of serenity that is your own private sanctuary.

Tips for Reducing Stress in Your Life

Certain hormonal changes triggered by stress can end up affecting the immune system, thus making us more susceptible to infections, and can also set off allergies, asthma, and rheumatoid arthritis. The release of extra sugars into the bloodstream can result in fatigue or hypoglycemia. The chronic tension and stiffness in the back that are characteristic of stress, especially when muscles are weakened by inactivity, lead to backache.

Stress can also cause:

~ Tingling and itchy skin, hives, difficulty in breathing, dizziness, and abdominal discomfort
~ Depressed sexual and reproductive functions, and an increase of premenstrual tension and menopausal melancholia
~ Depression, anxiety, and irritability

Stress is caused not only by bad events. Positive changes like a new home, marriage, and a new job can induce stress as well. Statisticians say that 9 out of 10 Americans report experiencing high levels of stress at least once or twice a week.

Stress-related disorders that were previously associated primarily with men are now on the rise in women. Stress leads to reduction in production of sex hormones in both men and women, and this can interfere with normal sexual functions. Stress causes increased muscle spasms, which are often responsible for lower back pain. Insomnia and other sleep disorders are very often the uncomfortable symptoms of a stress-related disorder.

Laughter is indeed good medicine. When you laugh, you actually cause a pleasurable change in your body's chemistry that lasts as long as 45 minutes. So take in a comedy at the movies, watch a funny television show, or invite some friends over for a game of charades!

Pets can provide excellent stress therapy. The presence of pets and physical contact with them has proved therapeutic for hospital patients. Play with your dog, hold your cat, or sing to your bird; all of these activities can help reduce blood pressure and bring a feeling of calm.

The soothing, stress-relieving power of nature has been recognized for centuries. Many hospitals and health centers now make "nature areas" a part of their therapeutic environment. When properly tailored to the individual's conditioning and enjoyment, exercise can help reduce stress and anxiety. Combine these two concepts by taking a walk outside, or try hiking, biking, or rowing.

Working at a desk for a prolonged period can increase tension and decrease efficiency. Concentration intensifies and each one of the five senses becomes more acute during stressful situations. But if taxed for too long, the senses become less acute. Doodling, a game of garbage-can basketball, or making paper-clip chains can provide a needed break and ultimately boost your productivity.

"Music hath charms to soothe a savage breast," wrote William Congreve back in 1697. Music's calming effect has been proved during dental procedures, labor, before and after surgery, and in emergency rooms. This is probably due to music's ability to distract and soothe. Similarly, while daydreaming is often criticized, it can provide a refreshing break from tension. It can be as simple as recalling pleasant memories or envisioning an upcoming vacation.

Remember that doing good feels good. Studies suggest that those who volunteer or do similar "good-neighbor" work have less incidence of stress-related disorders than those who do not perform such work. The benefits to health of human contact and companionship cannot be underestimated. Scientific research has revealed lower mortality rates in those with the strongest social ties.

Some causes of stress can be confronted and conquered. Others can be avoided. If you can't fight or flee, go with the flow.

Symptoms of Stress

These are the physical symptoms you're likely to feel when under stress:

~ Nervousness or inability to concentrate
~ Muscle tension and irritability
~ Heart palpitations or chest pain
~ Dry mouth or excessive sweating
~ Urge for under- or overeating, or loss of sex drive
~ Insomnia

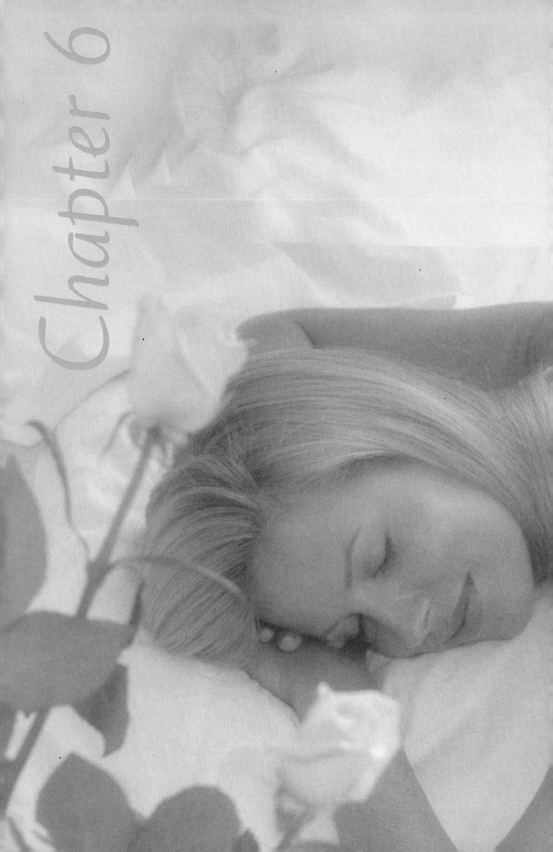

Chapter 6

the Sleep Soundly Bath

*S*leep 1: the natural periodic suspension of consciousness during which the powers of the body are restored
— *Merriam Webster's Collegiate Dictionary,* Tenth Edition

According to the American Institute of Preventive Medicine, more than 100 million Americans are estimated to have trouble sleeping, and 40 million Americans suffer from insomnia, whether it's a problem falling asleep or just staying asleep. But our bodies need sleep. It goes beyond being just a time of rest; sleep is a period during which physiological changes take place in our brains and bodies. Our metabolism and hormone production are reset and the immune system is bolstered. Sleeplessness, which disrupts these restorative functions, arises from complex mental and emotional issues.

When to See a Doctor

Good sleep is absolutely essential to good health. Compare proper sleep to a tune-up: Your batteries are recharged and your hormones are replenished. When we awaken from a good night's sleep, we are revitalized and rejuvenated. If you're a chronic insomniac, you may want to consult a healthcare professional who can help you determine the causes of your insomnia.

Insomnia, the most common sleep complaint, is the feeling that you have not slept well or long enough. It occurs in many different forms. Most often it is characterized by difficulty falling asleep (taking more than 30 to 45 minutes), awakening frequently during the night, or waking up early and being unable to get back to sleep.

Insomnia can begin at any age, and it can last for a few days (transient insomnia), a few weeks (short-term insomnia), or indefinitely (long-term insomnia). With rare exceptions, insomnia is a symptom of a problem and not the problem itself.

Long-Term Prevention for Insomnia

Stress is the most common cause of chronic insomnia. It isn't how much stress you have in your life, but how you handle it. Chronically tense people are frequently so restless and apprehensive that they *expect* not to sleep.

We all face a variety of stresses in our daily lives. While some people cope quite well, others have negative reactions — both physical and emotional — that not only disturb and disrupt sleep but also have an impact on their general health and well-being. Frustration and irritability are just the tip of the iceberg. The repercussions from a lack of sleep include serious traffic accidents, industrial accidents, high medical costs, and sick leave. Victims of sleep deprivation can actually suffer from opportunistic infections, depression, and anxiety.

In order to unravel the potential source of a sleep disturbance, you might want to ask yourself why an event stirs up a negative response. What are the thoughts that are scrambling around in your mind? What is not allowing you to welcome sleep? Becoming aware of negative ways that you respond to stress and to difficult situations is the first important step toward stress management.

Examine your soul and the emotions that are stirring inside of you. Examine the attitudes you hold about life. When we try to push issues out of our consciousness, they intrude on our inner consciousness.

SLEEP SOUNDLY BLEND

To quiet the mind and body in preparation for sleep, try this blend. If you are pregnant or asthmatic, skip the bath but do the accompanying meditation.

3 drops marjoram essential oil

2 drops lavender essential oil

2 drops sandalwood essential oil

1 drop ylang ylang essential oil

meditation exercise
Sleep Soundly

Light a blue candle for this exercise. Place the candle near the tub, but a safe distance from anything that could ignite (towels, shower curtains, tissues, for example). You will also need a watch with a second hand or a stopwatch.

Lie in the bath in a comfortable position, with your legs apart and relaxed so that your knees and hips are opened outward. Your head should be resting against the back of the tub. Lie there a few moments and see if you can keep your body absolutely still without becoming rigid with tension. Try to stay very still for up to 3 minutes. If you find yourself becoming tense or fidgety, take nice deep breaths, hold, and release slowly. With practice, your ability to become still will improve.

Look at the watch for 2 minutes. Try not to think of anything for those 2 minutes. Concentrate not on following your thoughts but only on registering them. If you find your mind traveling after a thought, stop the watch. Clear your mind; try not to think about anything. This may prove to be a more difficult exercise than you expected it to be; you may become aware of just how often your mind tends to wander. Repeat the exercise until you can do the entire 2 minutes without losing your concentration. Then relax in the tub, luxuriating as long as you desire until you are ready to do the visualization.

Now remove yourself from the bath and retire to your bedroom. Once under the covers, close your eyes and select an object that embodies the color blue, whether it be a flower, a sky, or a blue jay. Try to make this image the single and absolute focus of your mind. Now silently communicate to your subconscious, "Sleep, sleep, sleep . . ."

Pleasant dreams!

Sleep Maintenance Tips

Here are some tricks to help you get to sleep — and to stay that way until morning.

~ Transform your bedroom into a tranquil place for rest and dreams. Reserve the bed for sleeping. Prohibit television from the bedroom, as it can overstimulate you.

~ Work with your natural cycle — when you're sleepy, it's bedtime — and maintain a regular sleep/wake schedule. Keep the room as cool as possible to encourage your body's natural drop in temperature throughout the night. Avoid sensory distractions, like noise and light; they disrupt production of melatonin, a hormone that is directly related to your sleep cycle. Keep the bedroom dark and quiet at night.

~ Avoid excessive napping, stimulants, and alcohol. Eat a nutritious diet and exercise regularly, and, start relaxing *before* bedtime.

~ Once in bed, imagine that two huge hands are placed over your entire skull. See them as they massage slowly, penetrating your head until they are resting on your brain. Imagine the fingers gently stroking and massaging your brain. Imagine different layers of your brain expanding and letting go of stress as the magic hands caress and rub away your tension spots.

~ Try to imagine that you are looking at a clothesline strung with hanging clothes. Allow this to fill your vision so that you cannot see anything else. Think of each of your thoughts as an item of clothing on this line. Now picture each item of clothing being removed from the line as you silently say, "Let go of this thought, put it away." As each item is removed your thoughts are allowed to float away, and your mind will be free to drift into sleep.

~ As you lay your head on the pillow, close your eyes and watch the darkness wash over you. Concentrate on your breathing for a while, listening to the sound of your breath entering and leaving your body. Finally, let your thoughts drift as you slip slowly and gently toward a deep, reviving sleep.

~ Keep your bedroom well ventilated. Open your window just a crack and slip under a down comforter. Use a buckwheat hull pillow; it keeps you cool and is good for your spine.

~ Just before going to bed, drink a glass of warm cow's milk. Milk contains the calming amino acid L-tryptophan and can help you fall asleep. Sweets and fruit juices, on the other hand, contain sugars and should be avoided.

~ If you find yourself awake during the night, don't turn on the lights: Just 15 minutes of exposure to bright light in the middle of the night can disrupt the melatonin levels in your body, making it even more difficult to fall back asleep.

Determining How Much Sleep You Need

Most adults sleep between 7 and 8 hours, but no one really knows how much sleep we need. Sleep duration varies widely. Age also contributes to changes in the ability to sleep continuously and soundly. A newborn infant may sleep 16 hours a day, an adolescent may sleep very deeply for 9 or 10 hours straight, while an elderly person may take daytime naps and then sleep only 5 hours a night.

To find out how much sleep you need, try to determine your own sleep pattern. You should feel sleepy about the same time every evening. If you frequently have trouble staying awake in the daytime, you may not be sleeping long or well enough. You are sleeping as much as you need if, during your waking hours, you are alert and have a sense of well-being.

~ The best way to get a good night's rest is to keep a regular schedule for sleeping. Go to bed about the same time every night, but only when you are tired. Set your alarm clock to awaken you about the same time every morning — including weekends and regardless of the amount of sleep you have had. If you have a poor night's sleep, don't linger in bed or oversleep the next day. If you awaken before it is time to rise, get out of bed and start your day. Most insomniacs stay in bed too long and get up too late in the morning. By establishing a regular wake-up time, you help solidify the biological rhythms that establish your periods of peak efficiency during the 24-hour day.

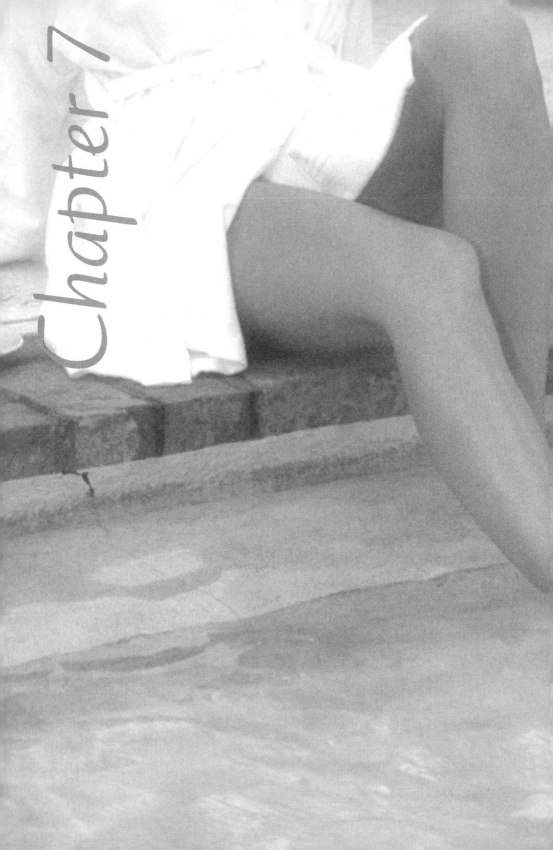

Chapter 7

the Revitalization Bath

The body can handle minor stress, but long-term stress causes the body to break down. Fatigue occurs when the situation that causes stress is not relieved. Find the cause and handle it constructively.

Your body is like your home: You need to maintain it. You cannot have a bright, cheerful home unless you let in lots of fresh air and sunshine; you must allow thoughts of joy and goodness to enter for a healthy body. Allow yourself time to enjoy time alone or with family and friends, try new things, and experience life in all its forms. Only then will the daily stresses wash away, leaving you refreshed and renewed.

Promote Well-Being from Inside

One of the secrets to a long life is to continue growing, reaching, and changing. If you are physically weak, start exercising your body. Jog, hike, swim, play tennis — do whatever physical activities you enjoy that will give your body the movement it needs. You can reap enormous benefits from even a small amount of physical activity every day. Dancing is one of the best workouts you can do, and is an excellent tonic for your spirits, too. It freely and joyfully enables you to let go of physical and mental tension. Setting aside times for daily relaxation is a good investment. It results in renewed energy and vigor.

If your thoughts are weak, start exercising your mind. Meditation and guided imagery are healthful and natural foods for your mind. Practice these regularly to strengthen your concentration and ability to deal with stress. Your mind is the key to healing, regeneration, and a healthy glow. If you desire a robust, energized, strong, healthy body, then think health and you will bring health and dissipate fatigue. Nourish your mind as you nourish your body.

Many leisure pursuits increase your mind and body's vitality, thereby aiding relaxation. Stake out frequent blocks of time to enjoy any hobby, from painting to gardening. Do the things you want to do and never feel guilty about taking time for yourself. Experiencing the happiness and satisfaction that come with pursuing a hobby is one of the best feelings you can have.

Once you establish the skills from exercising your mind and body, the desired effect can come about in even a very short time. It all depends on how much you are willing to put into it.

A period of deep relaxation before a trying time can set you up, giving you a boost of energy before a large expenditure. Similarly, a period of deep relaxation after a stressful time will renew and replenish your physical and mental resources. Never put off your relaxation time, thinking you can do it tomorrow. Start today, and enjoy the many benefits for years to come.

REVITALIZATION BLEND

To wake up in the morning, refresh you after a hard day's work, or before an evening out, this bath gives vitality to the physical body. If you are pregnant or asthmatic, do not use the bath but perform the accompanying visualization.

3   drops rosemary essential oil

2   drops peppermint essential oil

2   drops thyme essential oil

2   drops bergamot essential oil

Revitalization

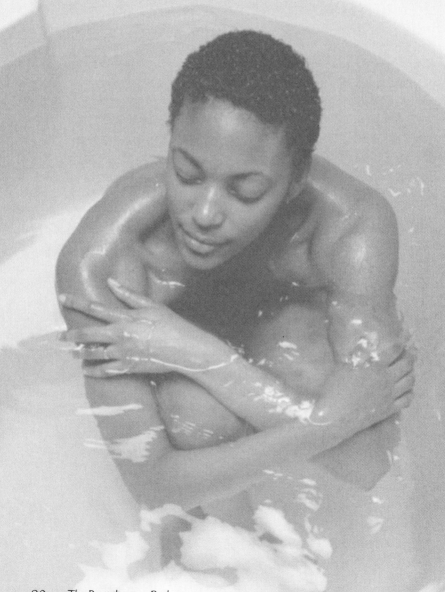

Light a yellow candle; place it where you can see it, but not near anything that could accidentally ignite. Climb into the bath.

Once in the bath, picture in your mind how blood circulates through the body. When it mixes with fresh oxygen, the blood is a vibrant, rich red color, but as it continues to travel farther from the lungs, it loses oxygen, and turns a darker shade of purple. Take a deep breath now and imagine that you are drawing in a massive amount of oxygen. As you exhale, you are blowing out useless carbon dioxide. Another deep breath invigorates the blood and draws oxygen deeper and deeper into the fatigued tissues. Take another breath, stretch, and see the oxygen reviving and replenishing all the blood cells in every fiber of your body. Breathe in again and see your body saturated with oxygen: vibrant, alive, and refreshed.

The golden yellow glow from the candle can nourish your soul, helping you regain your personal power and find your inner radiance. Envision this golden yellow as a bright sun sending you energizing rays, enveloping you as it wraps itself around you. Feel it restore and renew you inside and out. Remain in the tub for at least 15 minutes. Emerge from the tub when ready and extinguish the candle.

Tips to Keep You Feeling Revitalized

Get yourself into a regular routine of performing revitalizing activities or exercises; they will help keep you feeling energetic on a daily basis. Try these tips:

~ Get sufficient rest and sleep, and set aside time to practice deep relaxation.

~ Build up your endurance with proper exercise.

~ Take a 5-minute "soother" (i.e., relax in an armchair and breathe deeply) before engaging in stressful activities.

~ Do as little as 20 minutes of aerobic exercise several times each week. Aerobic exercise allows endorphins — a chemical that has been called "the brain's narcotic" — to be released into the system. Endorphins let your mind soar free and keep you feeling good for up to 5 hours after exercise.

~ Eat nutritious meals and develop your knowledge of vitamins and herbs.

~ Form a mental image of yourself as you intend to be. You will feel healthy, happy, and energized. Enjoy this picture and keep it foremost in your mind.

~ Use the Revitalization Blend as a morning booster. Add spring water to the recipe, then pour it into a spray bottle and lightly mist your body after you step out of the shower.

The following tips were shared by my dearest friend and workshop co-leader Reverend Charmaine Colón, Director of the Center for Spiritual Clarity and Development in New York and New Jersey:

~ Run your hands under cold water for about 20 seconds; it will give you a refreshed feeling and a sense of balance.

~ Breathe in deeply through the mouth and exhale the sound "ha." This will help release stress if done for 2 to 3 minutes.

~ Oftentimes, sharing our troubles with a friend will give us the pick-me-up we need to feel happy and enthusiastic about life. Your body knows it and shows it.

Case Study

I had a patient named Holly who was referred to me because of her depression. She was tired all the time and couldn't figure out the cause. After all, she had her own apartment, earned a great salary, was able to pay off school loans, and had good friends.

Holly was a good hypnotic subject and during that first hypnosis session we walked through her entire day from the minute she awoke. She was fine up until she visualized herself one block from her job. Becoming noticeably uncomfortable as she saw herself approaching the office door, Holly swallowed harder and verbalized that she felt a nausea rising to her throat. As she saw herself walking into her office, she burst into tears. In her conscious state, Holly did not realize that she had such a violent emotional and physical reaction to her job and workplace. She has since switched jobs and despite a small pay cut, she loves her work, has color in her face, and is very animated. She uses meditation and essential oils for "happiness maintenance," as she calls it, and is more revitalized now than she ever felt.

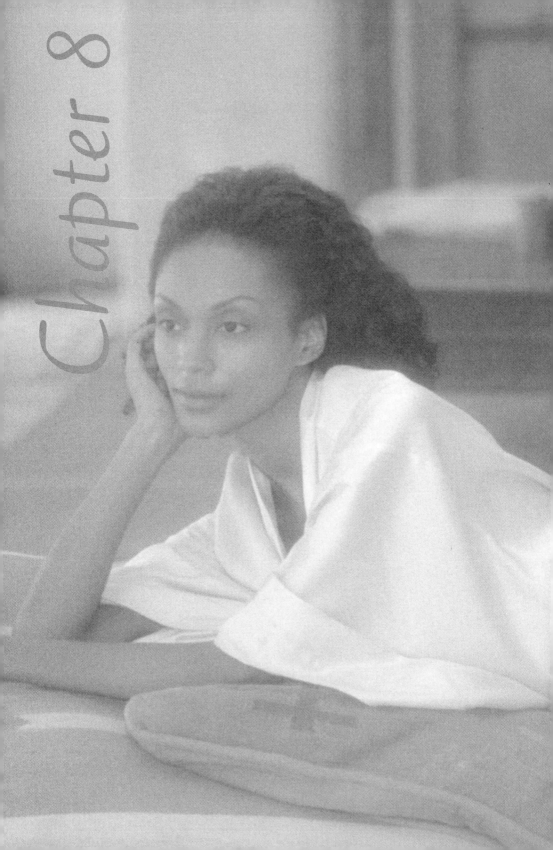

Chapter 8

the
Happiness
and
Harmony
Bath

*A*ccording to *Webster's,* happiness is "1: good fortune; 2: a state of well-being and contentment; 3: a pleasurable satisfaction." Harmony is "1: tuneful sound; 3: a pleasing or congruent arrangement of parts; internal calm."

Stop for a moment and evaluate where and how much you feel happiness and harmony in your life. Bringing awareness to it will bring it into your life on a day-to-day basis. Whether fleetingly or full flow, you will not allow moments of joy to slip through your day unnoticed and ignored. Everyone desires something — whether it's emotional, mental, physical, or spiritual. We all don't want the same things; some may want only enough to get by. Happiness means different things to different people at different times of their lives.

Tapping into Happiness and Harmony

When do you feel most alive? Is it when you fall in love? When you see a sunset? When you listen to your favorite music? I want you to visualize a special moment in your life that brought you happiness and joy. Close your eyes and take a few minutes. Open your eyes now. You can feel that feeling more often than you realize.

Give yourself permission to feel happiness without fear. However life is unfolding for you right now, there is within you some unknown source — a level of peacefulness with joy — that is beginning to express and expand itself. Experience the shift you feel when you change your perspective. You can access an enormous source of power.

Happiness is a condition of thinking as well, but being in the moment is an experience that you should give yourself permission to have more of. Look forward to these times daily, hour to hour, moment to moment. Happiness and harmony are achieved in the way you respond to each and every day without focusing on the frustrations in your life. Change your perception when problems arise.

Remember: "Mind over matter." Your mind is a powerful tool; use it to overcome any problems or obstacles or turmoil. Have faith in yourself and your abilities, and don't impose limitations. By examining your attitude about life, you can change negative perspectives to positive ones. For example, let's say that you're brooding because you're home alone on a Saturday night. You can let yourself sink deeper into that "pity party" or change your perspective to a positive one that says, "Well, I've got time to pamper myself, watch TV in the nude, or run to the nearest bookstore and buy an exciting novel to cuddle up with in bed."

Acknowledge and feel grateful about what you have in your life and you will create enthusiasm for your future. Each day is a fresh beginning. Many people know little joy in life, and until joy is discovered, it is difficult to proceed very far on the spiritual path.

I reiterate that happiness is an attitude of mind, born from your determination to be happy under all outward circumstances. Happiness does not lie in things or in attachments. It is the beauty of our inner nature buried beneath the "muck" of outward cravings. When you know that nothing outside can harm you — no disappointment, no failure, no misunderstanding from others — then you will know that you have found true happiness!

HAPPINESS AND HARMONY BLEND

This blend is good for when spirits are low and you are feeling depressed. If you are pregnant or asthmatic, skip the bath and proceed to the following visualization.

>   3   drops bergamot essential oil
>   3   drops ylang ylang essential oil
>   2   drops neroli essential oil
>   2   drops clary sage essential oil

Happiness & Harmony

Light a pink candle where you can see it (but a safe distance from flammable objects) or place a pink lightbulb into the bathroom fixture. Disperse the Happiness and Harmony bath blend in the bathwater. Once immersed in the bath, inhale the sweet, refreshing, fruity aromas of bergamot, ylang ylang, neroli, and clary sage, if using. Do some deep breathing until you feel your body relax.

In this visualization, you will use the color pink. This color is uplifting and relaxing, and should be used to encourage love and nurturing. Pink light is especially useful when you are feeling sad and lonely, unloved, rejected, or grieving. It provides much healing and nurturing of the emotions and connects you with universal love vibrations.

Stare at the pink candle without blinking, and when you can no longer hold your eyes open, allow them to close, bringing that pink color into your inner vision. Place your hands over your heart and allow the color to permeate your heart and chest area. See yourself receiving what it is you most desire that would make you happy and harmonious within yourself. See youself giving and receiving unconditional love.

Concentrate, focus, and visualize strongly. Visualize the pink flame burning in your heart and repeat inwardly, then outwardly, the following affirmation: "I will be happy and harmonious under any and every circumstance. I am love. I am joy. I am forgiving."

Emerge from the tub when ready and extinguish the candle. After your bath, pull on a pink T-shirt, nightgown, or nightshirt, or sleep on a bed dressed with pink sheets and pillowcases. The following day, wear the same color close to your body.

Tips for Encouraging Happiness and Harmony

~ Stretch out and increase alertness before getting up. Start stretching your body while sitting on the edge of the bed. Roll your head in a circular motion, allowing it to fall forward, to the side, and back. Stand up with your arms toward the ceiling, fingers outstretched, and reach first on one side, then the other. Now hang your head and arms loosely toward the floor and allow gravity to pull you down slowly. Stretch your spine while trying to touch your toes, and hang in that position for a while.

~ Take time for breakfast. Breakfast is a source of energy that you need to replenish blood glucose levels in the brain.

~ At night, create a peaceful, soothing, relaxing atmosphere in your bedroom by lighting candles and spritzing the specified essential oils throughout the room. Take care to extinguish all your candles before going to sleep.

~ Visualize a positive and creative day ahead of you, and think of all the good things you have in your life. Look forward to the good things that are coming your way.

~ Get sufficient rest and sleep. Eat well-balanced meals, and get regular exercise.

~ Blood sugars may dip in the afternoon, leading to a drop in energy levels, which can cause irritability, poor concentration, and lethargy. A small snack such as fresh fruit or some raw vegetables will provide a healthy pick-me-up in the afternoon. Eating fruit will supply a steady amount of glucose to your bloodstream, which in turn fuels your brain.

~ When people you love are pulling you in two directions, take a "time out" for yourself. Sitting quietly, tune out everyone else and follow your heart.

~ Buy yourself some flowers. Studies have shown that flowers reduce tension, discourage negative energy, and lift the spirits.

Case Study

Regina came into therapy with me a few years ago. She was 32 years old, hadn't been in a relationship for about eight years, and was still bitter and extremely angry at the hand life had dealt her. She lost her temper frequently and didn't last long in employment. Everything was everybody else's fault, everybody was against her. She had low self-esteem and got angry when people even looked her way. If Regina saw couples holding hands in the street, she would let that annoy her. She complained about not getting asked out on dates, but didn't realize that she was the one who kept people at bay.

The first few hypnosis inductions were for anger release. Regina listened to the taped induction from our session every night for two weeks and did the Anger Release Bath (see chapter 13) every other night. When she returned to me, she seemed much lighter, emotionally and even in physical movement. The next step was for her to choose to have happiness in her life. She did the happiness and harmony visualization for three weeks to great results. Regina calls every now and then to check in with me and sounds like a new person who is finally seeing and feeling what is good in this life. She also carries the Happiness and Harmony bath blend in a spray bottle in her purse!

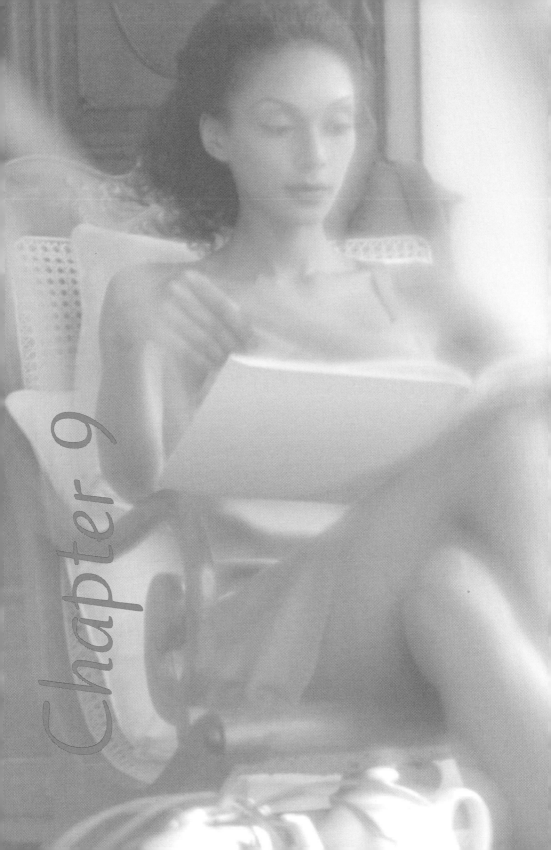

Chapter 9

the
Mental
Clarity
Bath

D o things seem to slip your mind? Do your thoughts wander or are you easily distracted? Is it difficult for you to concentrate on what you are doing? Does your mind feel like it's in a fog? Sometimes the harder you try to concentrate, the more difficult it is, and the more frustrated you become. The visualization and affirmation combined with the potent Mental Clarity blend will clear your mind and refresh it.

The Importance of Clarity

By improving your mental clarity, you improve your memory and ability to concentrate. Concentration can have an enormous impact on your everyday life. It makes you release your long-held dreams into reality; as Plato said, "We become what we contemplate." Jesus Christ spoke the truth when he said, "As a man thinketh, so he is."

Concentration is sustained attention. This means keeping your mind on one thing, to the exclusion of everything else. The more focused you are, the more you will exist in the moment, and you will no longer think about concentrating but, rather, simply experience it. With a clear, focused mind you can learn and retain more information in shorter amounts of time; this is particularly useful for students who would like to speed up their learning and earn better grades. Even when you eat a meal, for example, your food can be digested more easily and quickly if you concentrate on eating and absorbing rather than another activity such as reading or watching television. People are enormously successful in nearly any activity when they involve themselves in it 100 percent. Just think of all those Olympic athletes who have won medals by truly putting their minds to the task at hand.

The brain is a magnificent "bio-computer," designed to process immense amounts of information from many sources. The more you focus, the better able you will be to recall details from memory. Anything we experience is mentally recorded, but only the more important incidents and experiences are subject to recall. This process is carried out at will, or sometimes as an association of ideas from "triggers." When we make a conscious effort to remember, the unconscious mind continues to search for more details even after the conscious mind has abandoned the effort. By improving your memory and concentration, you will increase your awareness and ability to think more clearly and creatively with less effort.

MENTAL CLARITY BLEND

Mental Clarity is a blend that stimulates both body and mind. It is invaluable if you are mentally fatigued by overwork but need to maintain a clear head in order to complete some pressing tasks. If you are pregnant or asthmatic, do not use the bath but do the accompanying visualization exercise.

- 3 drops clary sage essential oil
- 3 drops rosemary
- 3 drops thyme
- 2 drops peppermint

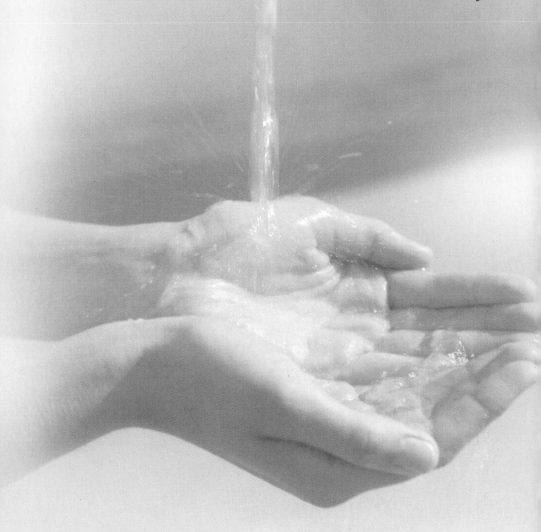

visualization exercise
Mental Clarity

Prepare the Mental Clarity bath blend and disperse it thoroughly in the bathwater. Light a deep blue candle and immerse yourself in the bath, deeply breathing in the aromas for about 3 minutes. With your eyes closed, allow yourself to focus on your breathing.

Allow any intruding thoughts to drift away. Imagine them floating on a cloud, or picture a helium balloon filled with these thoughts and watch the balloon drift off until you can no longer see it. Empty your mind and let all thoughts drift away without holding on to them.

Now picture yourself under a cool, refreshing waterfall that feels good on your body. Feel it cleansing your head and brain thoroughly. Any negative thoughts wash away from you; the coolness of the water sharpens your mind and body.

Visualize a strong deep blue ray of light from above. Walk into it, allowing it to permeate you. Let that color be the last thing you see and feel as you open your eyes.

Tips for Focusing the Mind

If you know how to focus and relax your mind, you will have an easier time practicing positive thinking. Most of the time you are using only part of your mental energies; your attention is subject to a thousand distractions and thus your thinking becomes cluttered and issues can seem more pressing than they really are. If you can learn to relax your mind as you relax your body, you can slow it down and allow yourself to exist calmly in the present.

Try some of the following suggestions for slowing down your thoughts, and you will start to discover greater perspective in your life. You also will improve both your memory and concentration. You'll enjoy using your mind to increase your awareness and you will think more clearly — and eventually with less effort. Focus on doing this right now before you are distracted!

Case Study

I once got a frantic call from Susan, who needed to see me immediately. She had been studying for an important exam on which hinged her hopes for a career change. As she studied so diligently, she experienced anxiety, loss of sleep, loss of appetite, and even loss of memory; she could not recall the answers she had worked so hard to memorize.

We had one session for improving study habits and concentration. At our next session, Susan visualized herself calmly taking the exam, effortlessly answering all the questions. Then she imagined herself excitedly receiving her excellent results. I gave Susan a small vial of the Mental Clarity bath blend, and she sprinkled a few drops on a handkerchief to sniff while she studied and took the exam. By using the blend coupled with mental techniques, Susan was able use the power of her mind to clear a successful pathway for herself. The following week we celebrated her passing the exam — she scored 98 percent on the oral portion and 100 percent on the written version!

Stop thinking! No one can stop thinking entirely; it is impossible. If you start trying not to think, you only end up thinking about how to stop thinking! What you can do, however, is to withdraw from your thoughts and become more of an objective spectator.

Picture your mind as a blank canvas or a dark sky. Allow your thoughts to come and go, but resist the urge to follow each one. Your brain will eventually slow down and you will feel less pressured.

Count. If you find it difficult to let go of your thoughts, try counting slowly as you breathe. Watch your thoughts and try to resist following them. Turn your attention to the count as you breathe out.

Pay active attention. As you work and think, try to keep your attention on the task at hand. Be strict with yourself, and each time your mind wanders, return it to the task. As you keep refocusing your attention, your "mind stillness" will improve.

Still your body. One sign of fragmented attention is fragmented movement. For example, when you are at the theater, it is easy to tell if others around you are fully attentive to the performance. People who sniff and sigh, move their heads this way and that, and wiggle in their seats are having some difficulty concentrating. Rapt attention is usually accompanied by still body posture.

Find a comfortable position and don't allow yourself to move. Concentrate on what you are doing or watching, drawing your attention away from physical distractions, and focus your thoughts on your task. After a while, you will notice that you fidget less and feel less physical discomfort. You are now channeled into mental exertion.

Interest your mind. Try to find interest in projects to help you concentrate. Taking up a new hobby can be a tremendous help. You should also try to find something interesting even in the dullest chore. If you are at a gathering, find someone and start a conversation. Be inquisitive and you might discover you have similar interests.

Open the mind. Just as strength, stamina, and flexibility must be incorporated in your physical routine, the mind needs new and absorbing challenges to give it a change from its everyday journeys.

Notice something new on the same way home that you might not have noticed before. Buy a magazine on a subject you normally wouldn't look at, read it, and open yourself up to new possibilities.

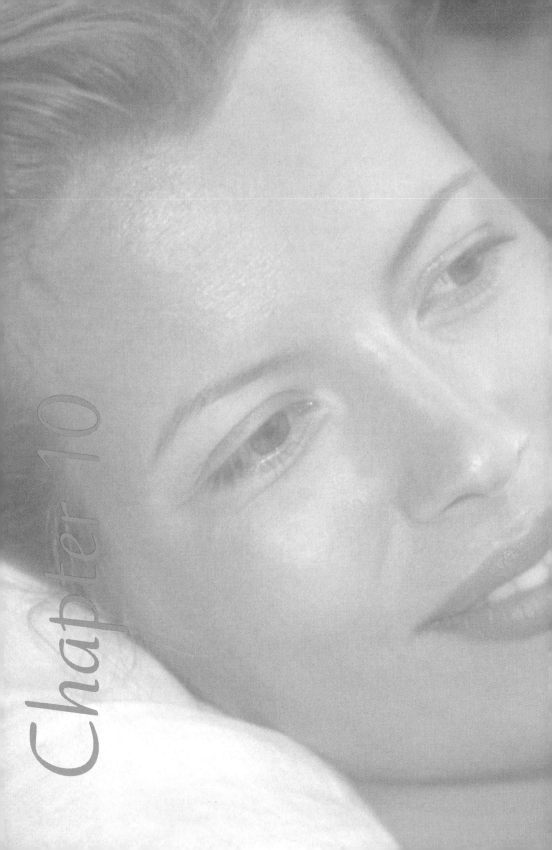

Chapter 10

the Love Bath

This complete bath cycle is to help heal and repair a broken heart. It facilitates the opening of your heart center, known in ayurvedic medicine as the heart chakra, to feel love for yourself first so that you can be more loving to others. When we truly love ourselves, we become love and it radiates throughout our entire beings. We then no longer have to think about loving others; we do it automatically.

Love is life's greatest blessing. We all need others; we need the emotional and spiritual nourishment of human relationships. Human comfort is a natural remedy for stress, tension, and doubt. Fear of the unknown, rejection, the loss of love, and criticism are major causes of loneliness. These very fears can create a vicious cycle of anger, boredom, or depression, which in turn creates more fear and isolation from others. But loneliness is a state of mind; the solution is to build bridges instead of walls.

The Chemistry of Love

Did you ever wonder what causes the feeling of "butterflies" in the stomach, or why you are perpetually happy when falling in love? Here is a look at the science behind what really makes us lose our hearts.

There are the four steps that help explain what happens biochemically when people fall head over heels in love.

1. The euphoria women and men feel when they first meet someone they are attracted to is the result of the brain releasing a chemical known as phenylethylamine, an amphetamine-like substance that is mildly hallucinogenic.

2. Next, the chemicals dopamine and norepinephrine are released in response to the phenylethylamine. These are the same chemicals the brain releases when we are fearful; they heighten our awareness of the world and may cause sweaty palms, heart palpitations, and increased breathing rate. The reason people eventually fall out

of this mad, helter-skelter stage is that just as a drug addict's body eventually develops a tolerance to dope, our bodies develop a tolerance to these naturally occurring brain chemicals.

3. The brain releases endorphins, the feel-good chemicals that make lovers feel comfortable and bonded and give them a feeling of security and peacefulness.

4. After lovemaking, the body releases the chemical oxytocin. Known as the "cuddle chemical," oxytocin is the same substance released when a woman nurses a baby. The chemical ensures that lovers feel connected.

Love and Healing

Learning to love yourself in healthy ways is the first step toward loving others. Seeing the beauty in you is as necessary as seeing the beauty in others. Create an atmosphere of love in your life. Your thoughts determine whom you attract into your world; concentrate on bringing more friendships, love, and beauty into your everyday life. Love is the source of all healing!

LOVE BATH BLEND

This blend aids in relaxation and expansive thoughts of love. It's also a good prelude for an intimate interlude! If you are pregnant or asthmatic, do not use the bath, but perform the accompanying visualization.

> 3 drops ylang ylang essential oil
>
> 2 drops clary sage essential oil
>
> 2 drops patchouli essential oil
>
> 2 drops neroli essential oil
>
> 1 drop rosemary essential oil

visualization exercise
Love
Visualization

Draw a bath and add the Love Bath
blend. Add 2 to 3 tablespoons of honey
and a few petals from a yellow rose to the
bathwater and mix well. Light a green
candle. (Green represents self-love and
trusting in the abundance of nature,
and will be used in the visualization.)
Look at yourself in a mirror.
Tell your reflection, "I love you . . . I
love you . . . I love you." Looking
deeply into your own eyes, feeling the connection, repeat out
loud, "I love you . . . I love you
. . . I love you . . . I love you."
Now step into the bath to begin
the journey.

Place your hands over your heart, close your eyes, and take a deep breath and hold it in. Wait a few moments, then release it. Begin letting your body relax, and continue to breathe in deeply. Breathe in again and hold it, then release and feel your body relaxing.

As you breathe in, imagine that you can breathe directly into the center of your heart. Inhale and feel your breath enter your heart center. Become more and more aware of your heart as you breathe. Inhale and imagine that you are breathing in a light of green. With each breath, experience the green light entering your heart, and allow a sense of warmth to enter as well. Sense a healing warm green light on your heart. Let the light illuminate places of darkness, tightness, and numbness. Keep drawing the light into your heart to fill your chest area.

Say a prayer inwardly, asking for healing. Ask for your heart to be open and healed. Imagine yourself being held, being cradled and rocked and loved, cuddled in your mother's arms. Breathe in, release, and receive.

Visualize a time in your life where you felt the most love. Remember those feelings and bring them into your heart. Feel the enveloping embrace of a loved one, feel the trust, gentleness, and vitality that blend with this feeling. Know now that you have remembered who you really are: a lovable person.

After the bath, stand in front of the mirror again and say aloud "I love you, I love you, I love you." Stay with that love energy.

Tips for Bringing Love into Your Life

Try these tips to make yourself feel more loved and loving in your daily life.

~ Every morning and night say "I love you" to your reflection.

~ Receive a long, long hug.

~ Hug your pet.

~ Prepare for love by speaking kindly to all you meet.

~ Consciously look for the good and positive in everyone.

~ Tell people of their finer points.

~ Begin to see more of the joy and beauty of life that is surrounding you daily.

~ Buy flowers for yourself and spread them throughout every room, including the bathroom.

~ Listen carefully to the words that others speak.

~ *Show* your love. Love is more than saying "I love you." It is saying it with your daily actions and the things you do — for example, by helping to cook dinner or being affectionate and understanding if your partner comes home late. Bake extra cookies and share them with a neighbor who lives alone.

~ Write down three ways in which you can give your love to others without expecting or needing anything in return. Select one of the ways and actually commit to sharing your love with someone today and tomorrow and the next day.

~ For one moment, let everything go from your mind. Right now, in this very instant, accept the joy that is yours for bringing love and light to others.

~ Pay a visit to someone ill.

~ Do some charity work for the elderly, hospitalized children, or homeless people in shelters. Donating your time, effort, and love of others will touch others' hearts.

Putting Love into Practice

In Manhattan, New York, there are many people rushing past, but one day I decided to brighten the day for other people. I bought a dozen roses, and when I saw someone with sad eyes, a frustrated look, or body language that said he was carrying the weight of the world on his shoulders, I gave him a rose and said quickly, "Have a nice day." I got some suspicious looks, but also several delighted thank-yous. After we arrived at my office, I gave the taxi driver a rose along with his tip. It woke him right up! He placed it on his dashboard so all his passengers could enjoy it as well. He seemed genuinely proud of it.

When I walked into my office I was charged with joy and love because my heart chakra was activated by what I did. My emotions overcame me several times. I was happy to have made others happy, if only for a fleeting moment, but the abundant feeling I had caught me off guard. When you give unconditionally, your own heart is filled and your love "runneth over."

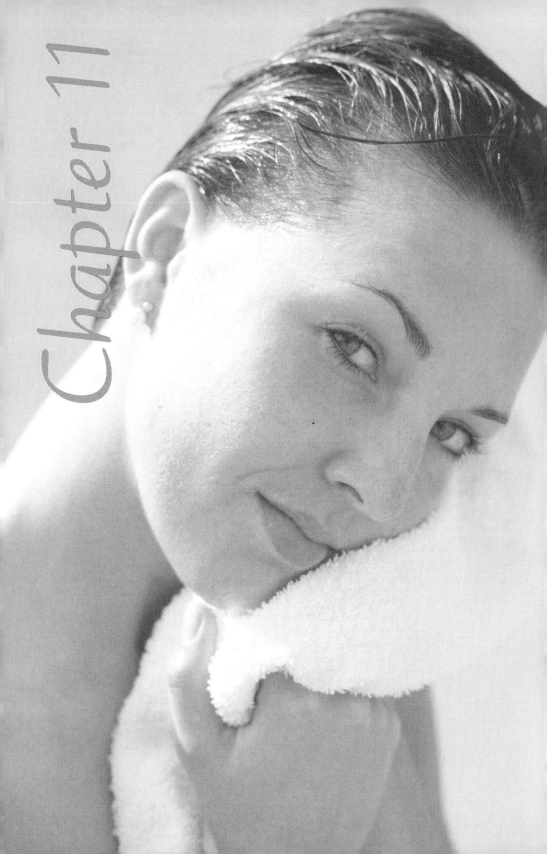

Chapter 11

the Increased Confidence Bath

Confidence comes from within. It's an inner strength and glow that radiates through in all you say, do, and feel. Self-confidence really develops from a feeling that you have some degree of control over your life's events (as much as anyone possibly can). You view life as an exciting challenge rather than an impending doom or threat. People who expect to succeed generally do; those who lack courage and constantly complain often fail. When you think about success, you become successful. When you think confidently, you become confident. You already have it within you; it just needs to be nurtured.

Changing Your Perspective

Lack of confidence can also come from negative programming that has adversely affected your development. Perhaps a parent put you down, or a teacher failed to recognize your assets and potential, or a demanding employer fired you. Maybe even some of your own actions are responsible, but you need to leave the past behind and not allow it to hold you back.

While you cannot make the events of the past disappear, you can change the perspective from which you view them — focusing on the positives instead of the negatives — to enable you to develop into the person you want to be. What you have assumed to be failure and accepted as failure were really learning experiences. Learning is essential to personal growth.

Suppose you got fired from a job that you thought held a sparkling future, and you got into a comfortable lifestyle. Maybe the dismissal was due to downsizing or a takeover, but it leaves you in a panic. You can either take it personally or learn from the experience. You can choose to take the skills you acquired there and tap into your survival instincts and move on. The saying is: "When a door closes, look for windows of opportunity."

You can transform "nervous energy" into positive energy. What may seem like nervousness is positive energy that you can consciously direct in any constructive way you want.

For example, if you're nervous about giving a presentation, recognize that you can use that energy productively. Begin focusing your mind either by meditating or writing down a detailed plan of action — how you want the presentation to go. Do some deep breathing to slow down. Understand that these nervous feelings can be transformed into good humor, an entertaining speech, or a mental quickness that will help you answer questions. Channel that energy productively instead of scattering it all over the place and getting nowhere.

If you have the need to grow, advance, improve, and move toward the achievement of your personal potential, this visualization will eliminate self-doubts and insecurities.

INCREASED CONFIDENCE BLEND

Increase your inner strength with this blend. You will think and become more confident! If you are pregnant or asthmatic, skip the bath and proceed to the following visualization.

> 3 drops clary sage essential oil
>
> 2 drops ylang ylang essential oil
>
> 3 drops myrrh essential oil
>
> 2 drops marjoram essential oil

Increased Confidence

Draw a bath and mix in the Increased Confidence blend. Light a blue candle (be sure the candle is not near anything that could accidentally catch fire) and climb into the tub. Breathe deeply and allow all your muscles to relax. Breathe deeply and take in the scents. With your eyes closed, visualize the color blue. Take another breath and allow your mind to daydream.

You are at a gathering of people, conversing. Visualize yourself relaxed and composed, speaking and acting with self-assurance, secure in your own knowledge. Now see and hear yourself saying, "I'm confident! I'm successful! I'm goal-oriented! I'm a winner!" Vividly picture yourself confident and full of inner strength. Focus all your thoughts on this image for as long as you can.

Now see yourself take new pride and joy in your growth and success with clear goals. For example, visualize yourself taking that night class that you've been putting off that can give you the freedom to move forward. Or perhaps you'd really like to ask for that raise you deserve. Maybe you can see yourself making that public presentation you feared more than anything and actually becoming excited about the opportunity.

Accept this suggestion deep into your subconscious mind, retaining it and believing it. By having allowed yourself to go into deep relaxation, focusing steadily and visualizing every detail of the desired outcome, you will bring it to fruition. Bring your awareness back to the present when ready.

Tips for Increasing Your Confidence

What can you do to promote the greatest degree of self-confidence when you're not in the bath? Here are a few suggestions:

~ Use your imagination as a positive force. Imagine only positive outcomes.
~ Visualize only scenes of success in your mind and look on the bright side. You have nothing to lose by being cheerful.
~ View life as an exciting challenge rather than as a threat.
~ Modify your response toward people you may find annoying.

If someone irritates you, don't stay around him or her longer than necessary. If it is in the workplace, excuse yourself, go to the privacy of your office or the bathroom, and do some "square breathing"; breathe in to the count of 4, release to the count of 4. Silently count to 4 before you breathe in again. Now that you have awareness, you have a choice of how to respond. You can also ignore a vexing person, keeping him from pulling you into his negative energy. He can disempower you only if you allow him to.

~ Learn how to reprogram your reactions to situations that arise. Find something positive that can come from the situation. Remember that you have a choice in the way you respond. See things from a different perspective; replace negative ideas with positive thoughts. If we think negative thoughts, we will attract negative thought forms; positive thoughts attract positive thought forms that beget the good things and people in our life.
~ Write affirmations of your own, carry them with you, and read them throughout the day.

Case Study

Nick finally came to me after canceling three appointments. It was his first therapy session and he was more than a tad nervous. When he walked into my office he was timid, looked down at the floor, and verbalized little. Although a survivor of a battered upbringing, he still had intact a very considerate and kind heart.

Nick shyly agreed to hypnosis sessions and it became a pleasant escape for him. In the sessions I diffused myrrh and thyme oils to help him increase his confidence level, move through obstacles such as past traumas, and revive and energize him.

Goals were set, and with some effort Nick would make eye contact or strike up a conversation with a stranger while waiting for the bus. Being aware of his body posture, he practiced social "courtship" skills and became more verbally expressive and less bashful. He started to make important changes in his life. Nick became more aware of his needs, stood up for himself more, and became an active, confident participant in his own life.

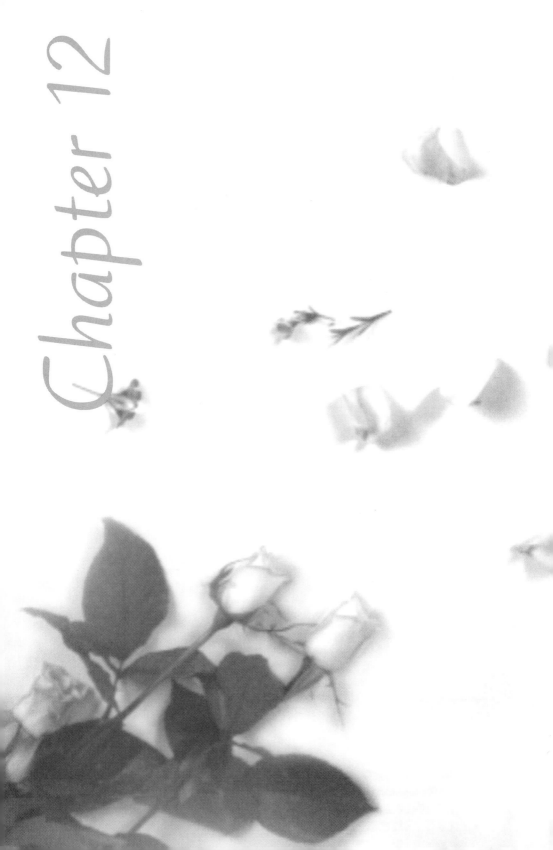

Chapter 12

the
Flower
Healing
Bath

*C*hakra is a Sanskrit word that means "wheel." The chakras are spinning vortexes of energy, the network through which body, mind, and spirit interact as a holistic system. By activating the seven chakras, you will release physical, mental, and spiritual blocks.

Energy created from our emotions and mental attitudes runs through the chakras and is distributed to our cells, tissues, and organs. By sending breath to the seven main chakra points, you open and charge each chakra and the surrounding organs with a vital life force. You direct breath to a chakra by focusing on the location of the chakra and visualizing the breath being sent to that area.

Chakras are doorways for our consciousness through which emotional, mental, and spiritual forces flow into physical expression. Each of these chakras is ascribed a dominant color and has a special link with

FLOWER HEALING BLEND

Flower healing is the most powerful way to open, activate, energize, and balance all of our chakras. Do not use the bath if you are pregnant or asthmatic, but perform the accompanying visualization.

3   drops ylang ylang essential oil
3   drops patchouli essential oil
2   drops myrrh essential oil
1   drop peppermint essential oil
2   drops sandalwood essential oil

A Guide to the Chakras

The seven chakras are defined as follows:

CHAKRA	LOCATION	COLOR*	PURPOSE
First (root)	base of the spine	red	Aids in your survival and how you interrelate with the world.
Second (navel)	just below the belly button	orange	Expresses the feeling of vitality and increases sex drive and creativity.
Third (solar plexus)	above the navel, just below the rib cage	yellow	Vitalizes the nervous system and gives self-assurance.
Fourth (heart)	center of the chest	green	Energizes the blood circulation. When this energy center is open, you feel compassion.
Fifth (throat)	throat area	blue	Facilitates communication.
Sixth (brow)	center of the forehead, between the eyebrows	indigo (dark blue)	Increases intuition and insight.
Seventh (crown)	top of the head	violet	Vitalizes the upper brain. You will feel a wonderful, joyous connection to everything and everyone around you. You will achieve great clarity and insight.

*for visualization

one of the endocrine glands and a physical organ. The colors are the seven colors of the rainbow spectrum. Each assigned color, when visualized with focused breathing, activates the energy in the chakra.

The Benefits of Flower Healing

The following bath visualization will consciously expand your experience of unconditional love, gratitude, compassion, forgiveness, and creativity. During this meditation, you will visualize a particular color corresponding to each chakra to balance that part of your body. You will bring yourself more harmony, creating a sense of wholeness within yourself.

Flower Healing

Prepare the bath and light a white candle. Place the candle near the tub, but safely out of reach of flammable materials. Accept its calming effects and spiritual qualities. Gather a small bunch of white carnations pulled from the stems and place them in the tub. Immerse yourself in the bath and begin to breathe deeply. Allow your eyes to close; take a deep breath and hold it for a few moments. Release and repeat. Imagine the white flowers that are floating around you.

Focus on the root chakra near the base of your spine. Imagine the color red as a spinning globe. Send your breath to that area and see it spinning, then opening up into a red flower. See the petals fluttering open. Focus on the area just below your navel; this is your second chakra. Visualize a spinning ball of orange. Now see it open up into a bright orange flower, and see the petals fluttering and opening.

Bring your attention up to your third chakra, above the navel. See a yellow, sunlike ball shining and spinning brightly, then imagine it opening up, petal by petal, into the brightest yellow flower.

Concentrate on the center of your chest, the fourth chakra. See a ball of green glowing and spinning. When it stops, the green leaves open slowly. What a wonderful feeling!

Focus on your fifth chakra, at the throat. Now visualize a globe of sky blue come into your throat spinning and becoming the loveliest flower. Watch as it opens up, petal by petal. Now concentrate on the "third eye" area in between your brows. A spinning ball of dark blue or indigo vibrantly glows and opens. Now all your attention should focus on the crown chakra at the top of your head. Visualize the color violet spinning and opening, releasing any pressure at the top of the head.

Now see all of the brilliant colors spinning. A white pure light of energy cleanses you from the bottom of your spine through all the colors and out the top of your head, and cascades down to your feet. You are cleansed and balanced! Your consciousness will come to full awareness now.

Tips for Maintaining Balance

The flower healing practice brings more understanding of yourself to you. By better understanding ourselves, we are able to make our choices and decisions from a place of awareness and balance.

To maintain this overall good feeling:

~ Live your life with integrity and honesty.

~ Eat fresh fruits and vegetables that are the corresponding colors of the chakras.

~ Fast for short periods (1 to 2 days); do this *only* under the supervision of a holistic doctor.

~ Try the chakra exercise while standing, placing your hands over each chakra point and bringing sound to each rapid breath while visualizing the assigned color. This helps clear emotional blocks.

~ Lie in bed and place gemstones or crystals with the corresponding color of each chakra on the naked body while visualizing the healing effects of each color. Allow yourself to absorb this energy, or allow the thoughts and images to surface on their own. If you find yourself getting impatient or tense, it means you are focusing too much on the technique and getting caught up in trying to do it right. Take a break, recover your sense of humor and playfulness, and begin the exercise again.

~ Put clear, clean quartz crystals in a pitcher of your drinking water. They help restructure the crystalline properties of the water and therefore help the activation and acceleration of personal consciousness.

~ Give of yourself unselfishly; selfless service will help to open the chakras in a natural and non-forceful way.

~ Make the time to walk in a beautiful place in nature.

~ Become more aware of your breathing; conscious breathing aligns the body, mind, and spirit.

~ Use your imagination. It is one of the most valuable tools that you possess for creating any reality you choose. Reality is what you dream it to be.

Making Floral Waters

Floral waters are refreshing and cleansing skin tonics. You can make your own floral water at home by adding 20 drops of essential oil to a 3½-ounce bottle of spring or distilled water. The best oils to use are essential oil of rose, orange blossom, and lavender, but feel free to try your own favorite — as long as you are aware of the oil's properties and are using it appropriately (refer to pages 41–49 for more information on the properties of essential oils). Leave the oil-and-water mixture in a dark place for a few days. Filter the oil from the water by using a large paper coffee filter. Apply with a cotton ball daily, preferably morning and night. Be sure to avoid the eye area.

Chapter 13

the Anger Release Bath

*A*nger is bad for your heart. When you blow up at somebody or something, you're putting tremendous added pressure and demands on your heart by making it pump harder, faster, and less efficiently. If you are prone to fits of temper, you are risking immediate and harmful changes in your heart. The secret is to cool it before your anger escalates. The emotion of anger stunts your spiritual growth, your creativity, and your vision. Directing your anger toward a positive outcome increases the healing potential of this process.

Why Anger Is So Destructive

Anger is a defense mechanism. Much of it is based on the fear of being or feeling vulnerable. But anger does not make you safe; it is not the way for you to create distance from another person.

It is not necessary to be angry with someone else or with yourself, although the actions of others can sometimes make us very angry. Attributing blame is a waste of energy that may not lead to solving the problem. Instead, take yourself to a quiet place to contemplate; there you will know how best to access your own feelings. Just recognizing your feelings and experiencing them may be all you want for a while. Also, by changing the vocabulary you use, you might find that you can influence the way you feel. Get into the habit of using objective rather than judgmental statements about yourself and others. For instance, if someone important to you criticizes you, don't think "I hate him/her!" or "he/she doesn't understand me." Rather, think "I will not retaliate; I will be silent so I can manifest peace," "I manifest the positive qualities of love, honesty, humility, and respect," or "I am a beautiful, radiant being. I am calm, patient, and intelligent."

If you cannot resolve a problem within yourself, communicate your needs to the person who is the source of this irritation and frustration. When you create distance between yourself and the person you're angry at because you fear being vulnerable, your anger doesn't get resolved and you don't move through it.

Maintain a sense of humor, especially during trying times. Have you noticed that people who are at ease and relaxed often don't take themselves too seriously? Get in touch with the absurdity that sometimes occurs in life, laugh, and diffuse the anger or distress. By resolving anger, you will create a new, healthy way of living. By minimizing this emotion, you can lead a happier life.

With the following visualization you can be in complete control of your emotions and promote only the good and healthy emotions; positive thoughts and reactions will be present in your conscious mind. You will be able to find what triggers your anger and then practice visualizing a similar situation while maintaining calm. Directing your anger toward a positive outcome increases the healing potential of this process. You will enter a place where you will be able to express unsaid thoughts and feelings so you can move forward in harmony, peace, and love.

ANGER RELEASE BLEND

This blend allows you to maintain control of your emotions and direct your anger toward a positive outcome. If you are pregnant or asthmatic, do not use the bath, but perform the accompanying visualization.

2 drops lavender essential oil
2 drops peppermint essential oil
2 drops myrrh essential oil

Anger Release

Light a magenta (red mixed with violet)
candle, place it within view of the tub
but away from flammable objects, and
prepare the bath. Ease into the tub.
Allow your eyes to close, and
breathe through your nose for a
count of 4. Exhale through the
mouth for 8 counts and relax.
Breathe in again, then
exhale slowly for 8 counts,
relaxing more each time.
See yourself in a sit-
uation where you lost
your temper in the
past. This time
see yourself in
control. You
no longer
respond with
anger. You
respond with

understanding and are calm. You no longer feel a need to retaliate.

You can now allow people to be themselves and allow them their own priorities. You no longer get angry because they do not agree with you. The only value someone else's opinion has is the value you give it, and you don't get angry because the opinion is different from yours. Anger is negative, and because you are in control of your own emotions, you choose to be positive. You will never again react with uncontrolled anger. Instead of becoming angry, you will see the other person's view. You react with understanding and care, and are calm; you react with positive thoughts and emotions.

Now fill your inner vision with the color magenta. On a physical and mental level, this color allows you to let go of ideas and thought patterns that are no longer right for you. You are in complete control of your emotions; only the good and healthy emotions, thoughts, and positive reactions are present in your conscious and subconscious mind. Keep this energy and bring your awareness back when ready.

When you are ready, repeat these affirmations:

~ "I am not my anger."

~ "No matter what someone says to me, it cannot reach the inner me."

~ "I need not defend with anger."

Tips for Releasing Anger

When you are angry, take three deep breaths and mentally step back from the situation that is triggering this response. Think about what is making you angry for a couple of minutes. Ask yourself if it's really worth it — is it really all that important? In this more "cooled-off" frame of mind, look at all your options. There's always an answer other than anger, and by choosing this alternative, you could be preventing a future heart attack.

Don't eat when you are angry. It is very common for people to try to suppress uncomfortable emotions by turning to "comfort foods" and tasty but unhealthy snacks. Food eaten in this way is likely to be improperly digested. Instead of eating, breathe deeply to relax your body. Then try to deal constructively with what is upsetting you.

Anger that is swallowed lodges inside the body and does a lot of damage; release is necessary. If you cannot express your feelings to the person directly involved in triggering this reaction, go to the mirror and talk to *that* person. Verbalize everything you are feeling. "I'm upset." "I'm angry." "I'm hurt." Go on and on until you have released the anger. Take a deep breath, still looking in the mirror, and ask yourself, "How can I change this?" If you change the belief system inside that creates this type of behavior, you will not need to respond or react in this manner any more. Accept the image of a positive experience or outcome.

If you feel the urge, bash a pillow, saying any words that come to mind. Alternatively, take yourself to a quiet place to contemplate. Project the existing situation on to your mental screen, then change the details until you feel that the outcome is the best that you can achieve.

Changing your vocabulary can influence the way you feel: The way to control your life is to control your choice of words and thoughts. Cut out of your vocabulary words like "ought," "must," "should." These are words that firmly place you in the passive role of someone who does not make his or her own decisions. For example, if your spouse comes home late one day, don't say, "I should not be angry with my spouse for coming home late"; instead, tell yourself, "I am no longer angry that my spouse came home late."

You might find that you are much more comfortable with words like "prefer," "choose," "wish," "want," "decide," rather than more definite ones such as "am" and "will." This is fine, as long as it helps you achieve the desired effect. In time you probably will become more comfortable with them. You might even decide to do something you find unpleasant, but the decision places you firmly in the active role. You will be able to tolerate any discomfort because it is your choice. In this way, you become empowered, not helpless.

Case Study

Sherri had been emotionally abused by her ex-husband. He was controlling, demeaning, and insulting. But Sherri finally divorced him and got on with her life, or so she thought.

Sherri came to me to develop her self-esteem and confidence. But what came up in sessions was her realization that she had never expressed her anger from her ex-husband's treatment. She sabotaged relationships without realizing why and then just stopped dating altogether. Sherri dealt with the anger release in self-hypnosis and did the bath blend every other day for one month. She has let go of the anger and is much more satisfied in her life. She feels stress-free, more in control of her life, and more self-assured. She is pleased with the skills she has incorporated into her life to handle anxiety. She meditates, uses essential oils, and does affirmations every morning to maintain her new outlook on life.

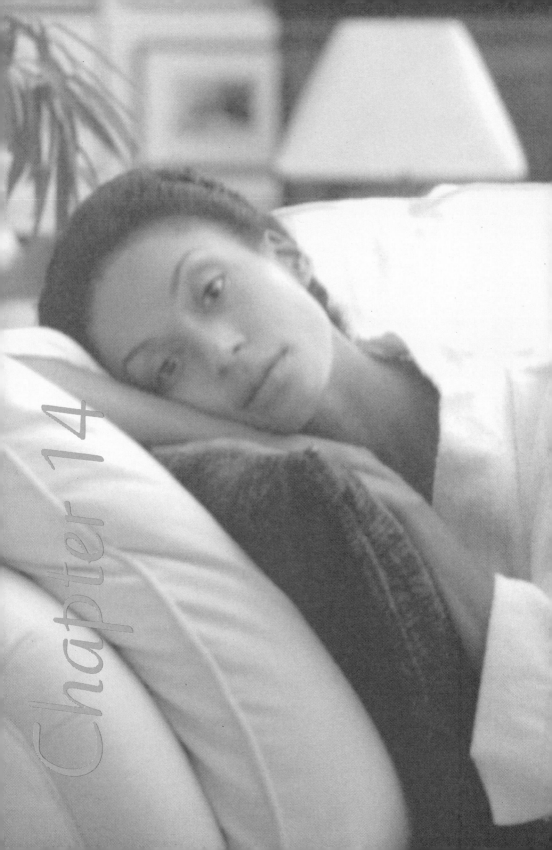

Chapter 14

the
Grief
Release
Bath

L et go of the pain.

Some people find that their lives are enriched if they allow themselves to have experiences in the here and now, without expending so much wasted energy on painful memories. They have no room for the "if only . . ." form of thinking. I am not suggesting that you block the past from your life; it is necessary to remember if you want to learn from that experience. But you should let go of the pain of past hurts. It is your choice, it is your experience.

Transform Your Emotions

Suppressing disruptive thoughts and feelings is not the way to transform them. Suppression causes your emotions to build up inside until enough pressure increases that, with little provocation, you explode and alienate friends and family. This can even lead to a breakdown. When your emotions are consumed with grief because of a great personal loss, feelings of bereavement, separation, and loss need to come to a closure so you are able to move forward in harmony, peace, and love.

By acknowledging that your spirit cannot be taken from you, that it is eternal, that death cannot steal it from us, you will take comfort in the fact that those we have known who have passed on are still here in pure spirit. Even though we won't be able to physically hold or hug them again, when it is time for us to leave our bodies, our spirits will again connect with theirs.

Be aware of whatever you need to grieve. If it causes you a lot of pain to think about the departed person, perhaps you didn't allow yourself to go through the mourning process; maybe you haven't completely expressed your feelings.

Everyone's grieving process is different; it is necessarry to evaluate the relationship and emotions that need to be addressed in your personal situation. It is also different with each person's loss that you grieve. Be aware of what your heart center is feeling. By your connection to this center, you will attain an awareness of what you need to do to express the emotions of loss, hurt, pain, or abandonment. Through awareness and expression you can experience renewal.

The absolute worst action you can take is repressing your thoughts and feelings. Some people believe this indicates moving on, when in reality it causes them to form mental blocks and become emotionally stagnant.

In this next imagery, you will embark on an inner journey and return with peacefulness, relaxation, and, most of all, acceptance. This will be a place to express unsaid thoughts and feelings to facilitate closure.

GRIEF RELEASE BLEND

This blend will assist you in letting go of the pain and finding closure. If you are pregnant or asthmatic, skip the bath and proceed to the following visualization.

2   drops ylang ylang essential oil

2   drops patchouli essential oil

2   drops marjoram essential oil

2   drops rosemary essential oil

visualization exercise
Grief Release

Light a red candle (red will dissolve grief and pain from the heart) and put it in a safe place within your view. Once in the bath, start off with a prayer that connects you with your Creator, or chant "om" over and over to connect you to your center. Inhale, then exhale and relax. Repeat several times.

Visualize a light streaming down from above, covering you from head to toe, bathing you completely within and without. This white light will protect and comfort you. It will keep you safe throughout this journey. Count backwards from 8 to 1, each number taking you deeper and deeper into a state of relaxation.

See yourself walking in nature, perhaps in a beautiful meadow with flowers swaying in a soft cool breeze. You keep walking until you see a bridge extended over cool, rushing blue water. The bridge is golden, majestic, and radiating. It is a magnificent sight. At the opposite end of the bridge, you see glittering shapes moving about. Allow yourself to recognize the person you wish to communicate with.

In the center of the bridge there is the cascading golden white light from above. You will walk to the center only and walk into this light. Do not go to the other side. The person coming toward you can come into the light to meet you but does not cross over to your side. Allow yourself to fully recognize the figure coming toward you in the light and make eye contact with him or her. Invite the person into the light in the center of the bridge. As you look into each other's eyes, say all the things you wished you had said before. Speak from your heart and soul.

Breathe in and out and allow all the deep sadness in your heart to fill you. The feeling might be a tightness in your chest, or an ache in your soul, or a swelling in your throat. Feel the pain deep in your heart. Breathe now into your heart as deeply as you can. Exhale — let it go! — releasing it in waves of tears or deep sobbing. Allow your grief and pain to express itself, then release it.

Now it is time to tell that person good-bye. Say it now, realizing you can both return to this place to visit and communicate. It is time to turn away and walk back. You turn, smile, and wave, and the person does the same. Your heart will be light as you continue off the bridge and walk back through the meadows. Affirm "I am free from suffering. I am at peace." Now say the phrase out loud.

Tips to Ease Your Grief

If you find that you're having a hard time letting go, understand that this is normal and nothing to be ashamed of. While it's true that time will lessen your grief, there are some activities you can do to facilitate the process.

~ See your breath as light, and direct it to various areas of the body. Expel darkness and pain through exhaling. The visualization is seeing the end result as you are totally healed, running through the fields.

~ Go to your place of worship, whether it is a church, temple, garden, or an altar at home, and pray and light candles in honor of the person you are grieving.

~ Meditate on those who have passed on, sending them thoughts of love and light.

~ Don't push away people who offer to help and support. Although you might feel that you want to be alone, companionship is an important part of healing.

~ When you're ready, open yourself to change. Spend time with close family and friends, or talk to your religious leader, a psychotherapist, or a counselor. Try some volunteer work or the arts to get you involved again. Self-help groups can be a tremendous support. Letter and journal writing are therapeutic, too. Take up gardening, cooking, or any other new skill you desire to learn. Plan a holiday, and allow yourself time simply to enjoy life.

~ Blend ½ ounce of jojoba or grapeseed oil with these essential oils: 1 drop ylang ylang, 1 drop clary sage, 1 drop marjoram, 2 drops rosemary, 2 drops rose. This mixture is very healing when rubbed on the abdomen in a steady, clockwise motion. It will facilitate the release of anger and sadness.

~ Have patience and faith. Try these helpful affirmations: "As I allow painful memories to surface, I know they are released and I am healed." "I am healed, balanced, and attuned physically, emotionally, mentally, and spiritually."

Case Study

Kenny walked into my office one year after his girlfriend committed suicide in their apartment. They had been having problems and his girlfriend had been using drugs that heavily contributed to her mood swings, irrational behavior, and paranoia. He'd had enough and planned to move out. One day, after visiting friends, he returned home to find she had taken her own life.

In the grief release hypnosis and aromatherapy sessions Kenny told his girlfriend what he didn't get to say before she died. Many painful bursts of emotions erupted from him with each induction. We also worked on releasing the anger he held for himself and his girlfriend, and then moved on to forgiveness: forgiving her, and forgiving himself for what he thought was his fault because he did not see it coming.

I am happy to say that Kenny has survived the experience, has a love and respect for life, and is now happily married. He even became a yoga and meditation instructor. He released his grief, his guilt, and his nightmares. I'm sure there will be moments of sadness when something reminds him of his painful experience, but it won't overcome him and he won't allow it to overshadow the happiness he has found.

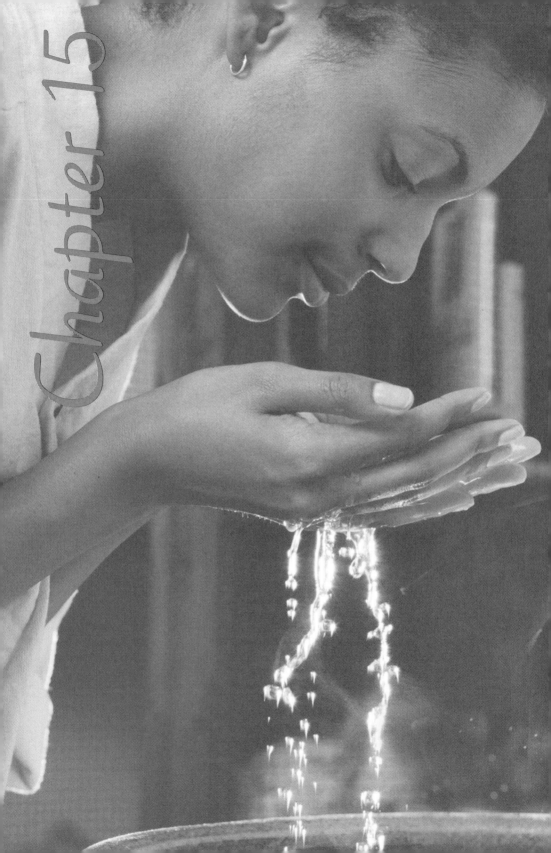

the
Forgiveness
Bath

To give up resentment against or the desire to punish an offender, you can find pardon — this is the process of forgiveness. By forgiving, you convert the suffering into psychological and spiritual growth. Forgiveness allows us to let go of some of our grief; when we have touched another with true forgiveness, we no longer require anything in return. It also benefits oneself and not just another; it brings about in us a new mercy and deeper understanding.

The Healing Power of Forgiveness

Forgiveness heals us and brings us deeper and closer to our hearts. All of us have a person or experience that we feel we will never forget and never forgive. When you refuse to forgive, you are holding onto the past, making it impossible to be fully in the present. When you are in the present, that is when you can create and manifest your future.

Case Study

Joan came to my weekly meditation healing circle and set up an appointment for private counseling. Her father had abandoned the family before she was born, and after her birth he made brief and infrequent appearances. He had multiple mistresses and always put down his children. One day Joan's father called her for the first time in 10 years to say he was dying. After some deliberation, she bought a plane ticket. He didn't even recognize her when she arrived. A week after his death she felt the need to let go and forgive him. Her anger was holding her back from being happy.

Joan was very receptive to hyponosis and aromatherapy, and we achieved wonderful results. She is empowered by not holding onto resentment or loss. She made the right decision, and is now able to live a more peaceful life.

You don't have to know a "secret recipe" for forgiveness; you just have to be willing. You can start by realizing that you don't want to hold onto negative and destructive emotions — you choose to let go and move on. Forgiveness is necessary for you even more so than for the person who hurt you. By forgiving yourself and others, you become free. Let go of the pain that holds you back. The weight will be lifted from your shoulders and you won't be bound by the past. When you come from love, you are safe. You will feel much lighter because you have freed yourself from that person or event.

Forgiveness should not be given mainly for its effects on others, but more for the freedom it reinforces in your own heart. You just have to be willing; if forgiveness doesn't flow from the moment, whatever is blocking forgiveness will become much clearer to you. To acknowledge the blockages of your heart is to open them to the healing that is needed. As you practice forgiveness, a new confidence arises within you. Forgiveness is a gift from your heart to your mind.

And by letting go of negative feelings and thoughts, your immune system gets stronger. By dwelling on negative emotions, we trigger physical reactions that use up our vital energy and weaken the body's immune system and our resistance to many diseases. Becoming a forgiving person will make you stronger, both mentally and physically.

FORGIVENESS BLEND

Use this blend to free yourself from anger and resentment. If you are are pregnant or asthmatic, do not use the bath, but perform the accompanying visualization.

- 2 drops peppermint essential oil
- 2 drops bergamot essential oil
- 2 drops myrrh essential oil
- 2 drops thyme essential oil

Forgiveness

Prepare the bath and light a dark blue candle. This will heighten your awareness of and sensitivity to beauty and love. Become nice and relaxed, breathing in the soothing scents. With your eyes closed, imagine emerald green healing energy bathing and enveloping your heart chakra (for an explanation of the heart chakra, see page 119).

Try to feel compassion and then forgiveness for yourself. Make a semi-fist (keep the thumb and the ring finger free) with your right hand and press your thumb gently against your right nostril. Exhale slowly through your left nostril. Then exhale through your right nostril, keeping your left nostril closed with your ring finger. Continue this breathing technique, altering nostrils, for about a minute. This breathing technique facilitates opening your heart chakra for a compassionate heart.

Inhale deeply and feel a strength come into your body; exhale your pain. Breathe in; as you exhale, release your fears. Take another deep breath; allow the powerful energy of love to fill your heart and lungs. Release the breath, feeling lighter now that the weight has been lifted.

Reflect on what the word "forgiveness" means. Bring into your mind the image of someone for whom you have harbored some resentment. Invite that person into your heart for that moment. Silently, in your heart, say to this person, "I forgive you." Feel his or her presence and say, "I forgive you for whatever pain you have caused me, however you may have caused me pain in the past. I forgive you." Repeat again, "I forgive you. I forgive you. I forgive you." Allow that person to continue sitting in the warmth and patience of your heart. Let him or her be forgiven. Bathe him or her in compassion.

Allow that person to go on his or her way with a blessing, taking as much time as you need. Now allow yourself back into your own heart. Allow yourself to be forgiven by you. Let the forgiveness fill your entire body. Allow yourself to be enveloped with love, kindness, and mercy. Embrace yourself with forgiveness and give yourself unconditional love. When you are ready, bring your awareness back and feel the lightness.

Tips to Help You Forgive

We all get angry and hold grudges from time to time, but these negative feeling are very unhealthy for both our physical and emotional well-being. To help you maintain your forgiving character, here are some tips.

~ Always forgive yourself for putting up with painful experiences, or not loving yourself enough to break away from those experiences. Holding a grudge against yourself will keep you from forgiving others.

~ Wear the color yellow to brighten your spirits.

~ Complete a yellow color visualization for a cleansing effect (see page 81 for directions). It will uplift you, bringing hope and light and a feeling that everything will work out. This exercise will dispel your fears and nervousness and help you develop personal power and the ability to value yourself more. It helps to stimulate mental clarity and open-mindedness, and helps in communication of thoughts. You will bring calmness to your mind and replace confusion with wisdom.

~ Alternate your yellow clothing with deep blue items; wear the color close to your skin and sleep on sheets of that color. Do blue color visualization for further healing. This color helps to raise your sensitivity and can be used for deep pain, healing, and purification. It brings clarity of vision. Deep blue helps you to take responsibility and direct your energy, your desires, and most importantly your thoughts to areas that will promote self-development and spiritual growth. It helps you to see the beauty all around you, and links you to your "higher mind" with intuition and the power of knowledge.

Resources

Is beauty a quality of the face, the body, or the spirit? Perhaps all three play a part, and if so, what better place of enhancement could you find than the bathtub? It is said that Cleopatra bathed in rose petals before she seduced Mark Anthony. Gypsy Rose Lee was known to contemplate her next conquest while bathing in essential oils.

Because the bath affords us a brief moment of tranquillity in our hectic lives, it is the perfect place to focus on being beautiful. Lie back in your tub and become aware of the beautiful fragrances that permeate your aura. This is a time for letting go. Let your body, mind, and soul drift to a new place of complete contentment. There is nothing else but the contemplation of your inner self.

Here are some excellent sources from which to purchase essential oils and blends for your aromatic healing bath.

AROMATICA, INC.
Margó Valentine Lazzara, C.Ht.
221 West 38th Street
New York, NY 10018
(800) BATH OIL; NY residents:
(718) 698-1616
Aromatica products draw from the history of the ages in developing harmonious fragrances that produce the most soothing baths. The complete collection of Aromatica Essential Oils for bathing is available through select retailers coast to coast, or order these products by phone. Hypnosis and aromatherapy consultations with Margó are available by appointment.

AURA-CACIA, INC.
P.O. Box 391
Weaverville, CA 96093
Write for a free catalog.

AUROMA
1007 West Webster
Chicago, IL 60614
(773) 248-1170
Fax: (773) 248-1174

AUROMA MELBOURNE
86 Burnwood Road
Hawthorn, Victoria 3122
AUSTRALIA
(03) 981-827673
Fax: (03) 981-183133

E'SCENTIALLY YOURS/THE
AROMATHERAPY PLACE
Pat Betty, aromatherapist and author
P.O. Box 909
New York, NY 10274
(212) 545-0229

ESSENTIALLY OILS
8-10 Mount Farm
Oxfordshire OX7-6NP
ENGLAND
011-44-0-1608-659-544

INDFRAG PRIVATE, LTD.
Philip Samuel
S-913 Manipal Centre
Dickenson Road
Bangalore 560 042 INDIA
081-258-9521

QUINTESSENCE AROMATHERAPY, INC.
P.O. Box 4996
Boulder, CO 80306
Write for a catalog.

MICHAEL SCHOLES
117 North Robertson Boulevard
Los Angeles, CA 90048
(310) 838-6122 or
(800) 677-2368
Fax: (310) 838-2812

RICHARD TAYLOR
Port of Spain, Trinidad
(809) 625-2580

WINDROSE AROMATICS
12629 North Tatum Boulevard,
Suite 611
Phoenix, AZ 85032
Write for a catalog.

Recommended Reading

Books

Allende, Isabel. *Aphrodite — A Memoir of the Senses.* New York: Harper Flamingo, 1998.
Anand, Margo. *The Art of Sexual Ecstasy.* Los Angeles: Jeremy Tarcher, Inc., 1989.
Austin, Milli. *The Healing Bath.* Rochester, VT: Healing Arts Press, 1997.
Cunningham, Scott. *Magical Aromatherapy.* St. Paul, MN: Llewellyn Publications, 1989.
Dodt, Colleen K. *The Essential Oils Book.* Pownal, VT: Storey Books, 1996.
The Fragrance Foundation. *Fragrance and Olfactory Dictionary and Directory.* New York: New York Fragrance Foundation, 1981.
Gawain, Shakti. *Creative Visualizations.* Novato, CA: New World Library, 1995.
Gindes, Bernard, M.D. *New Concepts of Hypnosis.* Hollywood, CA: Wilshire Book Co., 1951.
Hanhnhat, Thich. *The Blooming of a Lotus.* Boston: Beacon Press, 1993.
Jones, Alex. *Creative Thought Remedies.* Marina Del Rey, CA: Devorss and Co., 1986.
Levine, Stephen. *Guided Meditations and Explorations.* New York: Doubleday, 1991.
Rose, Jeanne. *The Aromatherapy Book.* Berkeley, CA: North Atlantic Books, 1990.
Valnet, Jean. *The Practice of Aromatherapy.* New York: Destiny Books, 1980.
Walters, Donald. *Affirmations for Self-Healing.* Santa Monica, CA: Crystal Clarity Publishers, 1990.

Magazines and Newsletters

Aromatherapy Quarterly
P.O. Box 421
Inverness, CA 94937-042
(415) 663-9519
Ask for information on the British version.

Aromatic Thymes
18-4 East Dyndee Road, Suite 200
Barrington, IL 60010
(847) 304-0975
Fax: (847) 304-0989

Index

Other Storey Titles You Will Enjoy

The Aromatherapy Companion, by Victoria H. Edwards. Prominent aromatherapist Victoria Edwards shares her 13 years of experience to create the most comprehensive aromatherapy guide available. Readers will find detailed profiles of dozens of essential oils, and instructions for blending and using them to enhance health and well-being through skin-care applications and inhalations. 288 pages. Paperback. ISBN 1-58017-150-8.

Creating Fairy Garden Fragrances, by Linda K. Gannon. This beautifully illustrated book explores the magical, aromatic world of herbs and flowers and provides recipes for richly scented, exotic potpourri blends. Along with each blend are fairy and herbal lore, poetry, stories about the seasons and the enchanted creatures of the garden, and gift-packaging ideas. 64 pages. Hardcover. ISBN 1-58017-076-5.

The Essential Oils Book, by Colleen K. Dodt. A rich resource on the many applications of aromatherapy and its uses in everyday life including aromas for the home, scents for business environments, and essences for the elderly. 160 pages. Paperback. ISBN 0-88266-913-3.

The Herbal Body Book, by Stephanie Tourles. Learn how to transform common herbs, fruits, and grains into safe, economical, and natural personal care items. Contains more than 100 recipes to make facial scrubs, hair rinses and shampoos, soaps, cleansing lotions, moisturizers, lip balms, toothpaste, powders, insect repellents, and more. 128 pages. Paperback. ISBN 0-88266-880-3.

The Herbal Home Spa, by Greta Breedlove. These easy-to-make recipes include facial steams, scrubs, masks, and lip balms; massage oils, baths, rubs, and wraps; hand, nail, and foot treatments; and shampoos, dyes, and conditioners. Relaxing bathing rituals and massage techniques are also covered. 208 pages. Paperback. ISBN 0-88266-005-6.

Making Herbal Dream Pillows, by Jim Long. A fragrant dream pillow tucked into a pillowcase is said to stimulate emotions and long-lost memories and produce vivid dreams that are exciting, relaxing, or creative. This lavishly illustrated book offers step-by-step instructions for creating 15 herbal dream blends and pillows for custom-made dreams. 64 pages. Hardcover. ISBN 1-58017-075-7.

Perfumes, Splashes, & Colognes, by Nancy M. Booth. A professional perfumer reveals her trade secrets for creating personalized scents and re-creating favorite perfumes using herbs, essential oils, and alcohol. 176 pages. Paperback. ISBN 0-88266-985-0.

These books and other Storey Books are available at your bookstore, farm store, garden center, or directly from Storey Books, Schoolhouse Road, Pownal, VT 05261, or by calling 1-800-441-5700. Or visit our Web site at www.storey.com.